AF794201

European School of Oncology

Monographs

Series Editor: U. Veronesi

L. Domellöf (Ed.)

Drug Delivery in Cancer Treatment II

Symptom Control, Cytokines, Chemotherapy

Springer-Verlag Berlin Heidelberg New York
London Paris Tokyo Hong Kong

Lennart Domellöf

Department of Surgery
Regional Hospital
70185 Örebro, Sweden

The European School of Oncology gratefully acknowledges sponsorship for the Task Force received from Pharmacia, originators and manufacturers of Port-A-Cath®, implantable drug delivery systems, CADD™, ambulatory infusion pumps, and Estracyt® and Sterecyt®, cytostatics.

ISBN-13:978-3-642-74711-3 e-ISBN-13:978-3-642-74709-0
DOI: 10.1007/978-3-642-74709-0

This work is subject to copyright. All rights are reserved, whether the whole or part of the material is concerned, specifically the rights of translation, reprinting, re-use of illustrations, recitation, broadcasting, reproduction on microfilms or in other ways, and storage in data banks. Duplication of this publication or parts thereof is only permitted under the provisions of the German Copyright Law of September 9, 1965, in its version of June 24, 1985, and a copyright fee must always be paid. Violations fall under the prosecution act of the German Copyright Law.

© Springer-Verlag Berlin Heidelberg 1989
Softcover reprint of the hardcover 1st edition 1989

The use of general descriptive names, registered names, trademarks, etc. in this publication does not imply, even in the absence of a specific statement, that such names are exempt from the relevant protective laws and regulations and therefore free for general use.

Product Liability: The publisher can give no guarantee for information about drug dosage and application thereof contained in this book. In every individual case the respective user must check its accuracy by consulting other pharmaceutical literature.

2123/3145-543210

Foreword

The European School of Oncology came into existence to respond to a need for information, education and training in the field of the diagnosis and treatment of cancer. There are two main reasons why such an initiative was considered necessary. Firstly, the teaching of oncology requires a rigorously multidisciplinary approach which is difficult for the Universities to put into practice since their system is mainly disciplinary orientated. Secondly, the rate of technological development that impinges on the diagnosis and treatment of cancer has been so rapid that it is not an easy task for medical faculties to adapt their curricula flexibly.

With its residential courses for organ pathologies and the seminars on new techniques (laser, monoclonal antibodies, imaging techniques etc.) or on the principal therapeutic controversies (conservative or mutilating surgery, primary or adjuvant chemotherapy, radiotherapy alone or integrated), it is the ambition of the European School of Oncology to fill a cultural and scientific gap and, thereby, create a bridge between the University and Industry and between these two and daily medical practice.

One of the more recent initiatives of ESO has been the institution of permanent study groups, also called task forces, where a limited number of leading experts are invited to meet once a year with the aim of defining the state of the art and possibly reaching a consensus on future developments in specific fields of oncology.

The ESO Monograph series was designed with the specific purpose of disseminating the results of these study group meetings, and providing concise and updated reviews of the topic discussed.

It was decided to keep the layout relatively simple, in order to restrict the costs and make the monographs available in the shortest possible time, thus overcoming a common problem in medical literature: that of the material being outdated even before publication.

UMBERTO VERONESI
Chairman, Scientific Committee
European School of Oncology

Table of Contents

Introduction

L. Domellöf

Department of Surgery, Örebro Medical Centre Hospital, Örebro, Sweden

This second European School of Oncology Monograph on Drug Delivery covers some major fields of theoretical and clinical importance that were only touched upon or even left aside at our first Task Force meeting. We now hope to share with the reader the basis for our stimulating discussions on new therapeutical modalities and to present a survey of the literature, thereby revealing at least one area of surprising ignorance. The latter is probably explained by a communication gap between the manufacturers of drugs and delivery systems and clinical researchers.

The first chapter of this monograph deals with pain control as an indispensable part of the supportive care of cancer patients. It is important to emphasise that many patients spend their last months and weeks of life in great discomfort, suffering, and disability, also mentally, depriving them of a decent quality of life. Only recently have we started to change the attitude in oncology by recognising the role of support provided by palliative care at home or in home-like settings, and to individualise analgesic dosages as well as prevent possible side effects. This requires close contact with the patient and simple evaluation systems to monitor the effects on the quality of life.

In the second chapter drug-drug and drug-plastic interactions are reviewed. The reason for including this topic was the fact that increasingly complex anticancer drug treatments are combining several cytostatics with a great variety of other drugs and delivery systems. As we suspected, the information in the literature was scarce or nonexistent. Nevertheless, from the available reports on the concomitant administration of different drugs, important changes in drug bioavailability were found. The drug-drug interactions affected absorption, distribution, metabolism, and elimination. Furthermore, major drug-plastic interactions were observed for a few studied anticancer agents. Thus the existing fragmentary information reveals a multitude of effects of pharmacodynamic relevance and an unacceptable lack of basic knowledge. The contribution that can be made by pharmacologists in this area is underlined.

Next follows a review of modern approaches to immunotherapy. The complex biological effects induced by cytokines and other factors (biological response modifiers, BRMs) on appetite, energy balance, body weight, and temperature are discussed. BRMs are effective in the normal metabolic interplay on the cellular level. With the advent of genetic engineering and with monoclonal antibody technology, pure preparations of these substances can now be produced. Several BRMs have been tried or are constantly under study in clinical trials. Thus it is important to focus on BRMs as a new generation of agents in future cancer treatment.

Intraarterial regional chemotherapy has been effective in some patients with cancer of the liver, head and neck, bladder, prostate, uterus, ovary, and lung, but also in bone and soft-tissue sarcomas, melanomas, and brain tumours. The theoretical aim is to achieve high local concentrations of the anticancer agent and to minimise systemic side effects. However, this is possible only if the drug has a high first-pass uptake. This and other factors are reviewed and the clinical rationale is discussed in the light of recent data from randomised controlled studies in hepatic arterial infusion (HAI).

This leads us to present the state of the art of arterial chemoembolisation. In patients with locally advanced liver cancer this treatment is intended to prolong the exposure time of the anticancer agent by reducing or blocking the tumour blood flow. Ideally, this would result in a greater cell kill, at least with some drugs (mitomycin C) in hypoxic versus oxic cells. The heterogeneity of the blood supply and the great variety of colloidal drug carriers (microspheres) are reviewed and judged against the requirements for an ideal drug carrier in regional therapy. Preclinical and clinical experiences are presented, especially for degradable albumin and starch (DSM, Spherex®) microspheres plus anticancer agents, and compared with drug in oil (Lipiodol) emulsions.

However, there are other interesting and complex research projects going on to optimise the treatment of hypoxic tumour cells. The heterogeneity in neoplastic cell clones was mentioned as one major therapeutic obstacle in our first monograph. This is due, among other factors, to the existence of oxic and chronically anoxic cell populations. The latter have a limited response to radio- and chemotherapy. Acutely hypoxic cells have a rapidly restored oxygen tension and metabolism. Some recent advances in the treatment of hypoxic cells are presented, e.g., the development of improved chemosensitisers, improved bioreductive drugs, and manipulation of tumour hypoxia with microspheres or vasoactive drugs. The possible role of multiparameter flow cytometry as a probe to identify hypoxic cells is also discussed.

Finally, we present the experiences of an ongoing home-care study of intraarterial or systemic chemotherapy. The results point to an important gain in quality of life as well as reduced treatment expenses, and also indicate future treatment strategies. This last chapter can be seen as a bridge to the third monograph, in which we are planning to discuss in more detail the home-care aspects of pain relief, nutritional support, and drug delivery to cancer patients.

Acknowledgements

On behalf of the Task Force, I would like to thank our active observers Pjotr Israëls, M.D. and Ria Dubbelman, R.N., for their valuable participation. We all acknowledge the excellent help of the E.S.O. staff in arranging the meeting and in preparing the monograph. We extend our thanks to Pharmacia for promoting this multidisciplinary monograph through their generous support.

Analgesic Drugs in Palliative Care

V. Ventafridda, A. Caraceni, A. Sbanotto, E. Spoldi, F. De Conno

Pain Therapy and Palliative Care Service, National Cancer Institute, Milan, Italy

Introduction

Palliative care consists of a new way of supporting the terminally ill who prove unresponsive to specific antitumor treatment to improve their quality of survival. By quality of survival we mean the psychosocial, environmental, and physical conditions of the individual which deteriorate during the advanced and terminal phases of cancer. It is a multidisciplinary approach, encompassing the patient, the family, and the community in its scope.

This is a new area of medicine that aims to counter the dehumanizing element still present in the intensive care of advanced cancer patients.

The primary goal of palliative care is the control of physical symptoms and, above all, of pain, within the context of continuing care up to the last moment of life.

Continuing care requires monitoring to be carried out by a team of specially trained therapeutic medical-nursing personnel working together with the patient's family at home, in the hospital unit, or in special homelike settings (hospice, palliative care unit, etc.).

The aim of this chapter, strictly based on the therapeutic issue, is to supplement the information contained in the previous monograph on the pharmacological treatment of pain [1]. The present chapter includes aspects of the monitoring of analgesics, the use of nonsteroid inflammatory drugs and an update on the administration of opioids.

Analgesic Drug Monitoring

One of the major topics currently under discussion in the research into pharmacological control of pain for cancer patients is the search for a quantifiable method of evaluating and monitoring analgesic response to drugs in order to:

1) predict the clinical effect;
2) administer appropriate chronic treatment and follow the patient's progress up to the last moment, outside the hospital environment;
3) conduct studies on pain and analgesia in chronic treatment. Problems here arise from the need to find some means of measuring the analgesic effect that reveals the changes caused by the drug [2].

Intensity scales of different types, including verbal categories and numeric and analog scales have been widely adopted for cancer-derived as well as other types of pain [3,4]. Such scales all give a one-dimensional evaluation of the symptomatology; in particular the visual analog has proved extremely sensitive to variations in pain intensity [5].

Houde et al. [5,7] and Beecher [8], using categorical and visual scales to measure the pharmacodynamic response, demonstrated the relationship between the dosage administered and the analgesic effect. In these studies, the average analgesic response in patients with pain varied with the logarithm of doses administered [6-9].

Among the instruments of evaluation, the McGill Pain Questionnaire provided a quantitative estimate that takes into account the multidimensional nature (sensory, emotional, affective) of each pain experience; national adaptations and modifications of this questionnaire represent an attempt to meet the need for comparison between results obtained in different countries by different authors [10-13]. Few attempts have been made, however, to use this or other methods to provide a classification that might allow a controlled study of the various pain syndromes typical of the advanced stages of cancer [14-19]. It is indeed well known that tumors may produce a variety of pain syndromes, depending on the pathogenesis or the semeiotic features of the case. In the individual patient these syndromes are often associated with a multiplicity of psychophysiological factors which together modify the symptomatology and response to treatment.

Recently an attempt has been made to provide a clinical staging of cancer patients with pain in order to identify the favorable and unfavorable prognoses for pharmacological treatment [20].

In the clinical practice of continuing care, there is a need to evaluate the analgesic effectiveness of pharmacological treatment and the changes that take place throughout the period of illness until death. Physical variables (the appearance of new types of pain, other symptoms), as well as social and emotional ones, determine clinical situations that require prompt assessment and control.

As regards research, it must be borne in mind that studies of analgesic drugs over short periods (6-8 hours) often give data quite different from those collected during prolonged observation. Monitoring is performed with quite simple means such as weekly self-descriptive forms, giving an overall evaluation of the patient's pain and general condition, and taking into account certain specific parameters:

1) Duration and intensity of pain for each day of the week;
2) The patient's activity (Performance Status or ECOG scale);
3) Symptoms other than pain;
4) Drugs taken and their daily dosages;
5) Indices of quality of life, expressing the quality of the patient's interpersonal and emotional life.

Forms like this permit a remote surveillance of the patient which is fundamental to the hospital teams providing follow-up at the patient's home. The Pain Therapy and Palliative Care Service at the National Cancer Institute in Milan has employed this kind of system to monitor thousands of patients over the years [21,22].

The forms used are preferably filled in by the patient with the help of a home nurse or family member; they provide invaluable information for the responsible team, which meets weekly at the hospital to decide any changes necessary to the therapeutic program. The computer-stored data can also be used to analyze the progress of the other clinical factors mentioned above. Other methods are also used, but in different therapeutic settings (e.g. hospitalized patients) [23,24].

A particular feature of pain evaluation is that of clinical-scientific research, which is more directed toward studying the relationships between pain and the biological characteristics of the patient.

As regards the relationship between analgesic effect and plasma concentration during treatment, and in relation to different forms of administration, no significant results have been obtained yet, partly because of the variable factors involved: some specific to the cause of the pain, others more general, e.g., age, race, intensity, site, and type of pain, and others again related to the method of administration used [25-31].

Of enormous importance in this area are pharmacokinetic studies that allow us to predict variability factors from patient to patient and to individualize treatment on the basis of the patient's pharmacokinetic characteristics [32-34]. Recent pharmacodynamic and pharmacokinetic models have enabled researchers to interpret the relationship between the plasma concentration of a drug and its analgesic effect; these factors partly explain the variability observed in the clinical use of such drugs [35-39].

It is essential for the clinician to use an instrument of evaluation both horizontally, in a continuous manner, and vertically, in discrete time periods; it should also be simple and not traumatic for the patient, whose only involvement should be to answer a few essential questions.

Nonsteroidal Antiinflammatory Drugs in Cancer Pain

As already mentioned in the previous monograph [1], nonsteroidal antiinflammatory drugs (NSAIDs) are the first choice for treatment of cancer pain and are used in scales II and III proposed by the WHO [40]. They are generally considered bland analgesics, but this definition is not adequate since in evaluating analgesic effects it is important to consider the nature of the pain as well as its intensity. In postoperative pain or oral surgery, antiinflammatory drugs may be superior to opioid analgesics [41]. The analgesic effect is linked to the blocking of the synthesis of prostaglandin by inhibiting cyclooxygenase [42,43]. Unlike opioids, NSAIDs do not modify sensory perceptions other than pain. They are, therefore, particularly useful in cases where inflammation is a dominant factor, for example in skeletal muscle pain [44].
Various authors have demonstrated a role of prostaglandins in the osteolytic activity of bone metastates. One of the primary indications for NSAIDs is still pain from bone metastases [44]. A retrospective study on 763 patients with cancer pain showed that the effectiveness of NSAIDs in chronic treatment as a single therapy was reduced by 25% by the fifth week. Furthermore, their action was reduced in neurogenic pain and by deafferentation [45].
However, various studies have shown that after about one month these drugs have no further effect, because of side effects in 50% of the patients and in the remaining 50% because of a lack of efficacy. A study on the pharmacological therapy of cancer pain following WHO guidelines showed that the average effective treatment time using NSAIDs alone was 19.2 days (± 24.5 SD) [46].

Drug Combinations

The rationale behind combining two or more analgesic drugs is based on the idea of acting on the mechanisms of analgesia at different levels. This, together with a desire to obtain the same results with smaller dosages and fewer side effects, has led, especially in the United States, to the use of analgesic compounds of NSAIDs and so-called minor narcotics. Studies performed show that the effect of optimal doses of two analgesic drugs in combination is given by adding the effects obtained with the two drugs alone. This was observed in various pain conditions: cancer pain [47,6] and oral surgery pain [41, 48]. The drugs concerned here were: acetaminophen, aspirin, oxycodon, codeine, and dextropropoxyphene. All these drugs showed an analgesic effect that can be significantly improved using an antiinflammatory drug and a narcotic, except for dextropropoxyphene which, with its long half-life, might accumulate in the plasma and is therefore more suitable for chronic clinical use than for controlled studies on single doses. For all the drugs, however, it was found that, in order to obtain a measurable effect, it was necessary to combine full dosages of NSAIDs (650-1,000 mg of acetaminophen or 650 mg of aspirin or the equivalent) with the usual dosage of narcotic [49].
These studies establish an extremely useful clinical principle and confirm the value of associating narcotic and anti-inflammatory drugs in the treatment of cancer pain. Combining several types of NSAID would appear useless because of the probability of increased side effects, with the exception of acetaminophen which has different undesirable effects from those of other drugs in this class.

NSAID Side Effects

The most serious clinical side effects in chronic NSAID treatment are gastrointestinal. It should be remembered that endoscopic lesions are found in nearly all cases where aspirin is administered to healthy volunteers. Chronic administration of 2.5 g of aspirin led to ulcers in 20% of cases, erosion of the mucous membrane in 40%, and "gastric erythema" in 75% [50]. Furthermore, there is no correlation between subjective symptomatology and the damage observed endoscopically [51]. One-third of the patients with known serious lesions were asymptomatic [50]. It should be noted that the impaired general condition of a patient with an advanced tumor undergoing chemo- and/or radiotherapy may contribute to gastric mucosal damage; other well-known risk factors are age, liver damage,

Table 1. Main mechanisms of NSAID damage

- Decrease of prostaglandin synthesis
- Increase of leukotriene synthesis
- Increase of oxygen metabolites
- Decrease of sulfydryls (glutathione)
- Local initiative effect

portal hypertension, and hemorrhagic diathesis. All the NSAIDs studied may provoke bleeding and damage to mucous membranes; the suggested mechanisms are listed in Table 1.

Endoscopically visible lesions were more readily induced with ibuprofen, sulindac, indometacine, naproxene, tolmetin, and aspirin than with a placebo [52]. In the light of these data, preventive measures should always be taken when giving chronic NSAID treatment. Ulcer medication with H2-blocking agents such as cimetidine and ranitidine has a proven protective effect on lesions produced by treatment with NSAIDs [53-55]. A protective effect of sucralfate was shown in three recent studies [56-58], but not confirmed in another [59]. This drug stimulates endogenic prostaglandin synthesis and has proved to be useful in the healing of already established lesions [60,61]. It is known that prostaglandins in doses of over 25 mcg are cytoprotective [60]. The following practical guidelines are recommended for the prevention of mucosal lesions and gastrointestinal bleeding caused by NSAIDs:

- use acetaminophen whenever possible, otherwise:
- combine with H2-blockers or sucralfate at the beginning of treatment;
- use enteric-coated preparations that are known to have fewer side effects, e.g. aspirin, ketoprofen, naproxene [51,62,63];
- avoid combination with potentially ulcerogenic high dosages of corticosteroids [64-72].

The risk of progressive renal failure when renal perfusion is threatened (cardiac failure, dehydration) may be prevented by careful monitoring of the indices of renal function in cases at risk [73].

Update on Opioid Analgesic Treatment

Morphine and related drugs exert their analgesic action on the opioid receptors at the level of the central nervous system. There has been some debate as to what extent the spinal and supraspinal sites of the opioid receptors contribute to the analgesic effect of morphine administered systemically or spinally [74,75]. However, it is clear that agonist opioids can produce analgesia by acting on the receptors at a spinal level [76,77].

The heterogeneous quality of these receptors is known and they are hence classified mu (mu1, mu2), delta, kappa, and epsilon receptors, with specific agonists and antagonists. Receptors mu, delta, and kappa are involved in spinal analgesia, but the various receptors seem to have different analgesic capacities in different experimental pain models [78]. This has led to a search for selective drugs with an analgesic mechanism unlike that of morphine (a global agonist), so as to limit side effects and overcome tolerance developed in one class of receptors. Experimental studies show that tolerance develops in all known receptors, but that there is no cross-tolerance between different classes of receptors [78]. Clinically, early experience with DADL (a delta receptor preferring agonist) administered intrathecally in patients tolerating opioids confirmed that the drug can have an analgesic effect but one that is not significantly different from morphine administered in the same way [79,80], however, in one case DADL reestablished analgesia in a patient tolerant to intrathecal morphine [81].

Many other neurotransmitters or modulators apart from opioids exert analgesic effects by acting on receptors at the spinal level, in particular noradrenaline, GABA, serotonin and acetylcholine. Clonidine (an alpha 2 agonist) was analgesic in patients with cancer pain when administered intrathecally [82] and peridurally [83]; in one case, the simultaneous administration of clonidine and hydromorphone gave better control of pain at lower dosages compared to increased dosages of hydromorphone [84].

These observations seem to confirm the experimental findings concerning interaction between the opioid and alpha adrenergic systems, which might produce a physiological analgesic effect with minimum activation of the respective receptor systems. Other interactions of this sort seem possible between baclofen and morphine, and between serotonin and noradrenaline [78]. Looking to the future, the side effects of single drugs might, therefore, be reduced and the development of tolerance modified.

A double-blind study comparing morphine and clonidine administered peridurally confirmed the usefulness of these drugs in the treatment of chronic pain, particularly where deafferentation was involved [85]. In all patients included in this study hypotension was observed, with a reduction of 20 mm Hg, as well as sedation, which was superior in patients receiving clonidine [150 mcg] compared with those receiving morphine (5 mg).

An important development is the discovery of effects such as hyperalgesia and dysesthesia induced by high intrathecal doses of morphine via a nonopioid mechanism [86]. If confirmed by clinical data, this would lead us to reconsider the possibility of raising dosages to very high levels in "tolerant" patients. One case is given of analgesia produced by a reduction in the dosage [86,87].

So far only one study has been able to demonstrate the advantages of spinal administration of analgesics over other methods. This study compared oral and spinal chronic administration of morphine to treat pain caused by cancer-induced lesions of the brachial or lumbar plexus [88]. It demonstrated that peridural administration was equally effective with a reduced incidence of side effects. It is true that nausea, vomiting, and sedation were also reported in the group undergoing peridural treatment.

Despite the very widespread use of these modifications and the development of more modern and sophisticated infusion techniques [89-93], there have been no controlled clinical studies to compare peridural, intrathecal, intravenous, and subcutaneous administration [94].

Although it has also been suggested that continuous infusion provides better control of pain and fewer side effects than periodic dosages, no studies have quantified the extent or significance of these occasional observations [95-97]. On the basis of the published data, it is impossible to give indications regarding peridural as against subarachnoidean procedures, or about the various technical options in the field, and still less concerning intraventricular techniques.

When adopting a rigorous protocol [95], one observes that some patients may benefit from spinal treatment in those cases where less invasive treatment has proven ineffective or problematic because of side effects. However, the success rate is very disappointing. Out of 24 patients using this method only 14 continued with the treatment after the test period and at least 6 of these had unsatisfactory results from long-term treatment. Thus only 30% of the patients benefited from this technique.

It would seem that the use of improved and technically perfect devices reduces the number of technical problems and has an overall positive impact on the result of therapy [88-90,95], but these studies still do not provide quantitative data about the real advantages of these types of administration.

Still less clear, from a clinical point of view, are the cases of intraventricular administration reported in the literature [98-100].

New Routes of Administration

In recent years there has been considerable interest in comparing transdermal administration methods with a growing number of drugs [101] and lately as a means of providing postoperative analgesia. With the administration of Fentanyl, pharmacokinetic studies have demonstrated the reliability of these transdermal systems with stable and constant plasma concentrations that compare favorably with those obtained intravenously [102-105]. The effectiveness and safety of this type of administration has been verified with postoperative pain scores [104-106] and seems to offer a very promising alternative to other forms of treatment, even in cases of chronic pain. Recently, a sample of 16 patients with cancer pain were treated using transdermal systems which can administer from 250 to 150 mg/h of Fentanyl and which are replaced every 3 days [107]. After having stabilized pain control with oral morphine, the symptoms were controlled for an average period of 84 days with a reduction in the consumption of morphine of between 180 and 90 mg. Further studies are necessary to assess the impor-

tance of these TTSs as a substitute for traditional administration.
Another form of parenteral administration that has received much attention is transnasal delivery which has been studied primarily in the antalgic field for Butorfanol, an agonist antagonist opioid, because of its small size and relatively lipophilic molecule. The effectiveness of this form of administration was claimed in an experimental study [108] and in various postoperative or postpartum pain trials where the appearance, intensity, and duration of analgesia (4 hours) were similar to those observed with intravenous administration [109-111]. It remains to be seen whether a role exists for this type of administration, perhaps it can be adopted with pure agonist drugs as rescue medication in patients chronically treated with opioids in other ways, thus avoiding the need for intramuscular or subcutaneous injections.

Patient-Controlled Analgesia (PCA)

Another form of analgesia that has received much attention is patient controlled analgesia (PCA), which has been evaluated intravenously or peridurally, especially for postoperative or other types of semi-chronic pain such as that caused by mucositis.
Two cases of PCA used to control tumor pain are reported [112,113], both in a hospital setting. A sample of 8 patients produced good analgesic results and satisfaction from the patients with a lock-out period of 90 minutes, intravenous doses of 2 to 5mg per bolus, at two-hourly intervals throughout the average study period of 28 hours. The authors recommend this method for short periods in patients with cancer-related pain [113]. To establish the validity of this treatment in the long run for outpatients, further studies are needed which compare other techniques already in use, such as continuous subcutaneous administration [97].
Faced with a symptomatology that contains a measurable element of stability, it would seem logical to propose symptom control using constant infusion systems, since parenteral methods are unavoidable. The usefulness of systems that permit programmed self-administration of extra boluses in controlled conditions is extremely interesting [1], both to allow rescue doses in the event of unstable symptoms and to compensate for varying plasma levels of the drug. Noncontrolled clinical experience with this type of treatment exists [114,115], but it requires further examination.

Morphine-6-Glucuronide

A recent discovery of interest is the analgesic effect of morphine metabolites, such as morphine-6-glucuronide (M6G) [116]. It is well known that the metabolite M6G has a powerful analgesic effect on rats when administered intraventricularly and overcomes the blood-brain barrier in this species [117]; in fact the effect is considerably greater than that of morphine itself.
In the chronic use of oral morphine the quantity of accumulated metabolite is extremely significant and varies considerably from individual to individual [118,119]. The effectiveness would seem to be attributable to the accumulation of metabolites, where M6G plays a fundamental part, and to the presence of the entero-hepatic cycle [116]. An early open study showed the effectiveness of intravenous M6G in 7 cases [120]. The results of oral administration in a limited number of patients are only preliminary, but promising.

Conclusions

Treating pain is only one part of the therapeutic approach and must not be separated either from the control of side effects or from the perception of the various physical and psychological symptoms that contribute to the patient's suffering in the advanced stages of cancer.
In the philosophy of palliative care, all analgesic treatments must be adapted to the individual patient and be sufficiently simple in their method of delivery to be used by the nurse, members of the family, and the patient himself. Our next monograph will cover the

therapeutic aspects of other methods of symptom control, as well as the modalities of applying palliative care at home and of coping with the psychosocial, emotional, and environmental problems.

REFERENCES

1 Ventafridda V, Sbanotto A, Spoldi E, Caraceni A and De Conno F: Cancer pain management and drug delivery. In: Domellof L (ed) Drug Delivery in Cancer Treatment. European School of Oncology Monograph Series,Springer-Verlag, Berlin 1987 pp 3-17

2 Colburn WA and Brazzell RK: Pharmacokinetics as an aid to understanding drug effects. In: Foley KM and Inturrisi CE (eds) Advances in Pain Research and Therapy. Vol 8. Raven Press, New York 1986 pp 427-440

3 Scott J and Huskisson EC: Graphic representation of pain. Pain 1976 (2):441-444

4 Deschamps M, Band PR and Coldman AJ: Assessment of adult cancer pain: shortcomings of current methods. Pain 1988 (32):133-139

5 Jensen MP, Karoly P and Braver S: The measurement of clinical pain intensity; a comparison of six methods. Pain 1986 (27):117-126

6 Houde RW, Wallenstein SL and Beaver WT: Clinical measurement of pain. In: De Stevens G (ed) Analgetics. Academic Press Inc, New York 1965 pp 75-127

7 Houde RW, Wallenstein SL and Rogers A: Clinical pharmacology of analgesics. 1. A method of assaying analgesic effect. Clin Pharmacol Ther 1960 (1):163-74

8 Beecher HK: The measurement of pain. In: Measurement of subjective responses. Oxford University Press Inc, New York 1959 pp 3-188

9 Beaver WT, Wallenstein SL, Houde RW and Rogers A: A clinical comparison of the analgesic effects of methadone and morphine administered intramuscularly and of orally and parenterally administered methadone. Clin Pharmacol Ther 1967 (8):415-426

10 Melzack R: The McGill Pain Questionnaire major properties and scoring methods. Pain 1975 (1):277-299

11 Bourlan F and Paquette C: Translated versus reconstructed McGill Pain Questionnaires: a comparative study of two French forms. In: Dubner R, Gebhart GF and Bond MR (eds) Proceedings of the Vth World Congress of Pain. Elsevier, Amsterdam 1988 pp 395-402

12 Maiani G and Sanavio E: Semantics of pain in Italy: the Italian version of the McGill Pain Questionnaire. Pain 1985 (22):399-405

13 De Benedittis G, Massei R, Nobili R and Pieri A: The Italian Pain Questionnaire. Pain 1988 (33):53-62

14 Ahles TA, Ruckdeschel JC and Blanchard EB: Cancer related pain - I. Prevalence in an outpatient setting as a function of stage and type of cancer. J Psychosom Res 1984 (28):121- 124

15 Graham C, Bond SS, Gerkovich MM and Cook MR: Use the McGill Pain Questionnaire in the assessment of cancer pain: replicability and consistency. Pain 1980 (8):377-387

16 Peteet J, Tay V, Cohen G and MacIntyre J: Pain characteristics and treatment in an outpatient cancer population. Cancer 1986 (57):1259-1265

17 Dent RL and Cleeland CS. The prevalence and severity of pain in cancer. Cancer 1982 (50):1913-1918

18 Cleeland CS, Ladinsky JL, Serbin RC and Thuy NC: Multidimensional measurement of cancer pain: comparison of US and Vietnamese patients. J Pain Sympt Manag 1988 (3):23- 27

19 Foley KM: Pain syndromes in patients with cancer. In: Bonica JJ and Ventafridda V (eds) Advances in Pain Research and Therapy. Vol 2. Raven Press, New York 1979 pp 59-75

20 Bruera E, MacMillan K, Hanson J and Mac Donald RN: The Edmonton staging system for cancer pain. J Pain Sympt Manag 1988 (3):521

21 Ventafridda V, De Conno F, Di Trapani P, Gallico S, Guarise G, Rigamonti G and Tamburini M: A new method of pain quantification based on a weekly self-descriptive record of the intensity and duration of pain. In: Bonica JJ, Lindblom V and Iggo A (eds) Advances in Pain Research and Therapy. Vol 5: Raven Press, New York 1983 pp 891-895

22 Tamburini M, Selmi S, De Conno F and Ventafridda V: Semantic descriptors of pain. Pain 1987 (25):187-193

23 Fishman B, Pasternack S, Wallenstein SL, Houde RW, Holland JC and Foley KM: The memorial pain assessment card. Cancer 1987 (60):1151-1158

24 Walker VA, Dicks B and Webb P: Pain assessment charts in the management of chronic cancer pain. Palliative Medicine 1987 (1):111-116

25 Ventafridda V, Ripamonti C, Lodi F, Saligari E, Panerai A, Gallucci M and De Conno F. Pain intensity: morphine and endorphine plasma levels during chronic administration of oral morphine. In: Foley KM and Inturrisi CE (eds) Advances in Pain Research and Therapy Vol 8. Raven Press, New York 1986 pp 95-102

26 Samuelsson H, Nordberg G, Hedner T and Lindqvist J: CSF and plasma morphine concentrations in cancer patients during chronic epidural morphine therapy and its relation to pain relief. Pain 1987 (30):303-310

27 Greene RF, Miser AW, Lester C, Balis FM and Poplack DG: Cerebrospinal fluid and plasma pharmacokinetics of morphine infusions in paediatric cancer patients and rhesus monkeys. Pain 1987 (30):339-348

28 Dahlstrom BE, Paalzow L, Segre LK and Agran AJ. Relation between morphine pharmacokinetics and analgesia. J Pharmacokinet Biopharmacol 1978 (6):41-53

29 Dahlstrom BE, Tamsen A, Paalzow L and Hartwig P: Patient controlled analgesic therapy I.V. Pharmacokinetics and analgesic plasma concentrations of morphine. Clin Pharmacokinet 1982 (7):266-279

30 Kaiko RF, Wallenstein SL, Rogers AG, Grabinski PY and Houde RW. Clinical analgesic studies and sources of variation in analgesic response to morphine. In: Foley M and Inturrisi CE (eds)

Advances in Pain Research and Therapy Vol 8. Raven Press, New York 1986 pp 13-23

31 Cousins MJ, Cherry DA and Gourlay GK: Acute and chronic pain use of spinal opioids. In: Cousins and Bridenbough PO (eds) Neural Blockade. Lippincott, Philadelphia 1988 pp 955-1029

32 Gourlay GK, Cherry DA and Cousins MJ: A comparative study of the efficacy and pharmacokinetics of oral methadone and morphine in the treatment of severe pain in patients with cancer. Pain 1986 (25):297-312

33 Plummer JL, Gourlay GK, Cherry DA and Cousins M: Estimation of methadone clearance: application in the management of cancer pain. Pain 1988 (33):313-322

34 Glynn C and Mather L: Clinical pharmacokinetics applied to patients with intractable pain: studies with pethidine. Pain 1982 (13):237-246

35 Perry J and Inturrisi CE. Analgesia and morphine disposition in burn patients. J Burn Care Rehab 1983 (4):276-279

36 Inturrisi CE, Colburn WA, Kaiko RF, Houde RW and Foley KM: Pharmacokinetics and pharmacodynamics of methadone in patients with chronic pain. Clin Pharmacol Ther 1987 (41)392-401

37 Inturrisi CE, Portenoy R, Max M, Stillman M, Colburn W and Foley KM: Pharmacokinetic-pharmacodynamic relationships of methadone and hydromorphone infusions in pain patients. J Pain Sympt Manag 1988 (3)S15

38 Inturrisi CE and Colburn WA: Application of pharmacokinetic- pharmacodynamic modeling to analysis. In: Foley KM and Inturrisi CE (eds) Advances in Pain Research and Therapy. Vol 8. Raven Press, New York, 1986 pp 441-452

39 Unadkat JD, Hill H and Walter MH: Does tolerance develop rapidly to the analgesic effect of alfentanyl? Clin Pharmacol Ther 1987 (41):181

40 World Health Organization: Cancer pain relief. WHO Office for publication, Geneva 1986

41 Cooper SA and Beaver WT: A model to evaluate mild analgesics in oral surgery outpatients. Clin Pharmacol Ther 1976 (20):241-250

42 Ferreira SH and Vane JR: New aspects of the mode of action of nonsteroidal antiinflammatory drugs. Annu Rev Pharmacol 1974 (14):57-73

43 Moncada S and Vane JR: Interactions between anti- inflammatory drugs and inflammatory mediators: a reference to products of arachidonic acid metabolism, Agent Action 1977 (3):141-148

44 Editorial: Osteolytic metastases. Lancet 1976 (2):1063-1064

45 Ventafridda V, Fochi C, De Conno F and Sganzerla E: Use of non-steroidal antiinflammatory drugs in the treatment of pain in cancer. Br J Clin Pharmacol 1980 (10):3435-3465

46 Ventafridda V, Tamburini M, Caraceni A, De Conno F and Naldi F: A validation study of the WHO method for cancer pain relief. Cancer 1987 (59):850-856

47 Moertel CG, Ahmann DL, Taylor WF et al: Relief of pain by oral medications: a controlled evaluation of analgesic combinations. JAMA 1974 (229):55-59

48 Cooper SA, Prenscheur H, Ranch D et al: Evaluation of oxycodone and acetaminophen in treatment of postoperative dental pain. Oral Surg 1980 (50):496-501

49 Beaver WT: Combination analgesics. Am J Med 1984 (77, 3A):38-53

50 Silvoso G, Ivey KJ, Butt et al: Incidence of gastric lesions in patients with rheumatic disease on chronic aspirin therapy. Ann Intern Med 1979 (91):517-520

51 Lanza FL: Endoscopic studies of gastric and duodenal injury after the use of ibuprofen, aspirin and other non-steroidal antiinflammatory agents. Am J Med 1984 (77):19-24

52 Butt JH, Barthel JS and Moore RA: Clinical spectrum of the upper gastrointestinal effects of non-steroidal antiinflammatory drugs. Am J Med 1988 (84,2A):5-13

53 Berkovitz J, Frank W, Kirsch T, Palmer R and Young MD: Effects of cimetidine on indomethacin-related mucosal damage. Gastroenterology 1987 (92):1914

54 Hoyan DL: Damage and protection of the human gastric mucosa. Am J Med 1988 (84,2A):35-40

55 Kimmey MB and Silverstein FE: Role of H2 receptor blockers in the prevention of gastric injury resulting from non- steroidal antiinflammatory agents. Am J Med 1988 (84,2A):49- 52

56 Danesh BJZ, Duncan A and Russell: Sucralfate (SF) protects against mucosal injury at a neutral gastric pH. Gastroenterology 1986 (90):1387

57 Konturek SJ, Kwiecian N, Kopp B and Olesky J. Double-blind controlled study on the effect of sucralfate on gastric prostaglandin formation and microbleeding in normal and aspirin treated humans. Gastroenterology 1986 (90):1499

58 Stern AI, Ward F, Hartley G. Sucralfate protects the human stomach from the damaging effect of aspirin. Gastroenterology 1986 (90):1648

59 Malchow-Moller, Ranlov PJ: Does sucralfate reduce acetylsalicilic-acid-induced gastric mucosal bleeding? Scand J Gastroenterol 1987 (22):550-552

60 Ivey KJ: Mechanisms of non-steroidal antiinflammatory drug- induced gastric damage. Am J Med 1988 (84 2A):41-48

61 Wu WC, Semble EL, Castell DO, Caldwell JR, Roth SH, Heller MD and Marsh WH: Chronic sucralfate therapy of non- steroidal anti-inflammatory drug induced gastritis: a multicenter trial. Gastroenterology 1986 (90):1696

62 Ryan JR, Riley WA, Vargas R, Offen WW and Gruber CM: Enteric coating of fenoprofen calcium reduces gastrointestinal microbleeding. Clin Pharmacol Ther 1987 (42):28-32

63 Trondstad RI, Aadland E, Holler T and Olanssen B: Gastroscopic findings after treatment with enteric-coated and plain naproxen tablets in healthy subjects. Scand J Gastroenterol 1985 (20):239-242

64 Conn HO and Blitzer BL: Nonassociation of adrenocorticosteroid therapy and peptic ulcer. N Engl J Med 1976 (294):473-479

65 Green B, Gail MH and Byar DP: Letter. N Engl J Med 1976 (294):1291
66 Long WB, Shiau Y: Letter. N Engl J Med 1976 (294):1291
67 Crass JR: Letter. N Engl J Med 1976 (294):1292
68 Sturdevant RAL: Letter. N Engl J Med 1976 (294):1292
69 Lubin A: Letter. N Engl J Med 1976 (294):1292
70 McDonald CJ: Letter. N Engl J Med 1976 (294):1292
71 Cooke AR: Letter. N Engl J Med 1976 (294):1292-1293
72 Conn HO and Blitzer BL: Letter. N Engl J Med 1976 (294):1293
73 Kantor TG: New strategies for the use of antiinflammatory agents. In: Dubner R, Gebhart GF and Bond MR (eds) Proceedings of the Vth World Congress on Pain. Elsevier, Amsterdam 1988 pp 80-86
74 Tang AM and Schoenfeld MJ: Comparison of subcutaneous and spinal subarachnoid injections of morphine on analgesic tests in the rat. Eur j Pharmacol 1978 (52):215-223
75 Clark SL, Edeson RO and Ryall RW: The relative significance of spinal and supraspinal actions in the antinociceptive effect of morphine in the dorsal horn: an evaluation of the microinjection technique. Br J Pharmac 1988 (79):807-818
76 Yaksh TL: Spinal opiate analgesia: characteristics and principles of action. Pain 1981 (11):293-346
77 Nordberg G: Pharmacokinetic aspects of spinal morphine analgesia. Acta Anaesthesiol Scan 1984, 28 (supp 79)
78 Yaksh TL and Stevens CW: Properties of the modulation of spinal nociceptive transmission by receptor-selective agents. In: Dubner R, Gebhart GF and Bond MR (eds) Proceedings of the Vth World Congress on Pain. Isevier, Amsterdam 1988 pp 417-435
79 Moulin D, Max MB, Kaiko RF, Inturrisi CE, Maggard J, Yaksh T and Foley KM: The analgesic efficacy of intrathecal D-Ala-D- Len-Enkephalin in cancer patients with chronic pain. Pain 1985 (23):213-221
80 Moulin DE, Inturrisi CE and Foley KM: Cerebrospinal fluid pharmacokinetics of D-Ala-DLen-Enkephalin. Ann Neurol 1986 (20):218-222
81 Kramer ES, Wilkie DJ and Gershaw J: Intrathecal D-Ala-D.len-Enkephalin (DADL) restores analgesia in a patient analgetically tolerant to intrathecal morphine sulphate. Pain 1986 (24):205-209
82 Coombs DW, Sanders R, Geylor M, La Chance D and Jensen L: Clinical trial of intrathecal clonidine for cancer pain. J Regional Anaesth 1984 (9):34-35
83 Germain H, Neron A and Lomssy A: Analgesic effect of epidural clonidine . In: Dubner R, Gebhart GF and Bond MR (eds Proceedings of the Vth World Congress on Pain. Elsevier, Amsterdam 1988 pp 473-476
84 Coombs DW, Saunders RL, Fratkin JD, Jensen LE and Murphy CA: Continuous intrathecal hydromorphone and clonidine for intractable cancer pain. J Neurosurg 1986 (64):890-894
85 Glynn C, Dawson D and Sanders R: A double blind comparison between epidural morphine and epidural clonidine in patients with chronic non-cancer pain. Pain 1988 (34):123-128
86 Yaksh TL, Harty GJ and Onofrio BM: High doses of spinal morphine produce a nonopiate receptor-mediated hyperesthesia: clinical and theoretic implications. Anesthesiology 1986 (64):590-597
87 Onofrio BM, Yaksh TL and Arnold LE: Continuous low-dose intrathecal morphine administration in the treatment of cronic pain of malignant origin. Mayo Clin Proc 1981 (56):516-520
88 Vainio A and Tigerstedt I: Opioid treatment for radiating cancer pain: oral administration vs. epidural morphine. Acta Anaesthesiol Scan 1988 (32):179-185
89 Yaksh TL and Onofrio BM: Retrospective consideration of the doses of morphine given intrathecally by chronic infusion in 163 patients by 19 physicians. Pain 1987 (31):211-223
90 Ventafridda V, Spoldi E, Caraceni A and De Conno F: Intraspinal morphine for cancer pain. Acta Anaesthesiol Scan 1987 (31, suppl 85):47-53
91 Penn R and Paice A: Chronic intrathecal morphine for intractable pain. J Neurosurg 1987 (67):182-186
92 Ingemar F, Ahlgren H and Ahlgren MBE: Epidural administration of opiates by a new device. Pain 1987 (31):353-357
93 Arner S, Rawal N and Gustafsson LL: Clinical experience of long-term treatment with epidural and intrathecal opioids - a nationwide survey. Acta Anaesthesiol Scan 1988 (32):253- 259
94 Cousins MJ: The spinal route of analgesia for acute and chronic pain. In: Dubner R, Gebhart GF and Bond MR (eds) Proceedings of the Vth World Congress on Pain, Elsevier, Amsterdam 1988 pp 454-476
95 Shetter AG, Hadley MN and Wilkinson E: Administration of intraspinal morphine sulfate for the treatment of intractable cancer pain. Neurosurgery 1986 (18):740-747
96 Ventafridda V, Spoldi E, Caraceni A, Tamburini M and De Conno F: The importance of continuous subcutaneous morphine administration for cancer pain control. The Pain Clinic 1986 (1):47-55
97 Bruera E, Brenneis C and MacDonald RN: Continuous Sc infusion of narcotics for the treatment of cancer pain: an update. Cancer Treat Rep 1987 (71):953-958
98 Obheus EAMT, Stratton Hill C, Leavens ME, Ruthenbeck SS and Otis F: Intraventricular morphine administration for control of chronic cancer pain. Pain 1987 (28):61-68
99 Lenzi A, Galli G, Gandolfini et al: Intraventricular morphine in paraneoplastic painful syndrome of the cervicofacial region. Experience in thirty-eight cases. J Neurosurg 1985 (17):6-11
100 Payne R: Novel routes of opioid administration in the management of cancer pain. Oncology April 1987 (special supplement)
101 Lasagna L and Greenblatt DJ: More than skin deep: transdermal drug delivery systems. N Engl J Med 1986 (314): 1638-1639
102 Kramer TH, Plezia PM, Lindford J and Hameroff SR: Pharmacokinetics of transdermally

administered fentanyl. Clin Pharmacol Ther 1987 (41):181
103 Nimmo WS and Duthie DJR: Plasma fentanyl concentrations after transdermal or IV infusion of fentanyl. Anaesthesiology 1986 (65)A559
104 Holley FO and Van Steennis C: Postoperative analgesia with fentanyl: pharmacokinetics and pharmacodynamics of costant- rate IV and transdermal delivery. Br J Anaesth 1988 (60):608-613
105 Duthie DJR, Rowbotham DJ, Wyld R, Henderson PD and Nimmo WS: Plasma fentanyl concentrations during transdermal delivery of fentanyl to surgical patients. Br J Anaesth 1988 (60):614-618
106 Oden RV, Caplan RC and Ready LB: Effect on ventilation of transdermal fentanyl compared to intramuscular morphine for postoperative analgesia following upper extremity orthopedic surgery. Pain 1987 (suppl 4):S156
107 Simmonds MA, Blain C, Richenbacher J and Southam MA: A new approach to the administration of opiates: TTS (Fentanyl) in the management of pain in patients with cancer. J Pain Sympt Manag 1988 (3):518
108 Suberg SN and Libera JM: Effect of intranasally (IN) administered butorphanol tartrate in the rat tail flick test. Pain 1987 (suppl 4):S155
109 Kurtz NM, Chu G and Abbond T: Intranasal butorphanol in postoperative pain. Pain 1987 (suppl 4):S153
110 Kurtz NM, Chu G, Cool M, Abbond T and Joyce TH: Analgesic efficacy and safety of intranasally administered butorphanol in post partum episiotomy pain. Pain 1987 (suppl 4):S153
111 Cool WM, Chu G, Kurtz N, Abbond T, Cooper S, Jain A, Joice T, McMahon G and Ryan J: Intranasal butorphanol: comparison of analgesic efficacy measures in different pain models. Clin Pharmacol Ther 1987 (41):162
112 Keeri-Szanto M: Demand analgesia for the relief of pain problems in terminal illness. Anesth Rev 1976:19-21
113 Citron ML, Johnston-Early A, Boyer M, Krasnow SH, Hood M and Cohen MH: Patient-controlled analgesia for severe cancer pain. Arch Intern Med 1986 (146):734-736
114 Kerr IG, Sone M, Ferris F, Coons C and Deangelis C: Outpatients continuous narcotic infusion with patient- controlled analgesia for chronic cancer pain. Abstract Book 3rd International Symposium The Pain Clinic, 1988 pp 176
115 Sone M, Kerr I, Wodinsky H, Ferris F, Coons , De Angelis C: An outpatient narcotic infusion programme for cancer pain; practical aspects. Abstract Book 3rd International Symposium The Pain Clinic, 1988 pp 176
116 Hanks GW, Aherne GW, Hoskin PJ, Turner P and Poulain P: Explanation for potency of repeated oral doses of morphine? Lancet 1987 (2):723-725
117 Yoshimura H, Ida S, Oguri K, Tsukamoto H: Biochemical basis for analgesic activity of morphine-6-glucuronide-I. Biochemical Pharmacol 1973 (22):1423-1430
118 Sawe J: High-dose morphine and methadone in cancer patients. Clinical pharmacokinetic considerations of oral treatment. Clinical Pharmacokinetics 1986 (11):87-106
119 McQuay H, Carroll D, Hunton J, Dutt S, Hand C and Moore A: Chronic cancer pain treated with morphine: plasma morphine and glucuronide metabolite (M3G and M6G) concentrations. J Pain Sympt Manag 1988 (3):S18
120 Osborne RJ, Joel S, Trew D and Slevin M: The pharmacologic activity and pharmacokinetics of intravenous Morphine-6- glucuronide in man. J Pain Sympt manag 1988 (3):S15

Pharmacokinetic Aspects of Drug-Drug and Drug-Plastic Interactions with Anticancer Drugs

Lennart K. Paalzow

Department of Biopharmaceutics and Pharmacokinetics, University of Uppsala, Uppsala, Sweden

Drug-Drug Interactions

In order to achieve an optimal cytotoxic effect on various neoplasms, the concurrent administration of several anticancer drugs with different mechanisms of action has become routine today. Clinical practice also shows that combination drug therapy often seems to be more effective than single drug treatment.

It should, however, be recognized that antineoplastic drugs are often pharmacodynamically very potent and many cytotoxic drugs exert their effects on rapidly proliferating cells in malignant tumors as well as in normal tissues (such as in bone marrow and intestinal mucosa). Therapeutic and toxic concentration ranges often overlap in treatments using several of these drugs. To avoid unnecessary toxic side effects with antineoplastic drugs, it is therefore important carefully to control the dosage, mode, and schedule of administration in order to achieve and maintain minimum effective concentration in cancer cells during optimal effective time. Thus, acquisition of the knowledge of the pharmacokinetic charateristics of anticancer drugs is an important tool in designing rational strategies for their clinical use. Unfortunately, experimental studies to define fundamental pharmacokinetic characteristics are still lacking for many drugs of this class.

In addition to multiple anticancer drug regimens, patients with neoplastic diseases often receive a variety of other drugs such as analgesics, sedatives, antiemetics, antibiotics, and so on. Thus, undesirable consequences of drug interactions may arise in many cases of cancer chemotherapy. To date, the main interest has been focused on pharmacodynamic interactions and their clinical significance; however, during the last years increasing attention has been paid to pharmacokinetic related drug-drug interactions [1].

In order to reach and maintain therapeutically effective concentrations in cancer cells, but also to minimize toxicity in normal tissues, it is important to consider interactions where the levels and duration of active substance in the body are affected by concurrent administration of other drugs. For instance, changes in the absorption, distribution, and elimination (biotransformation and excretion) of one drug can alter the biophase concentration and half-life of a second agent.

In the present review, some of the clinically most important pharmacokinetic related interactions of anticancer drugs and their possible kinetic explanations will be discussed. The drugs will be classified according to the level of the physiological process at which they will interact, i.e., at the steps of drug absorption, distribution, and elimination.

Absorption

Absorptive Process and Gastric Emptying

Cytostatic drugs are known to affect the rapidly proliferating epithelium of the gastrointestinal mucosa. The degree of inhibition of the intestinal mucosal regeneration depends on dose and duration of drug action and, in addition to the inhibition of cell renewal, cytostatic drugs have a toxic effect on epithelial cells. Morphological and functional alterations of the intestinal mucosa develop rapidly and are about the same for all cytostatic drugs [2].

An increasing number of elderly patients receive cancer chemotherapy and many of these drugs induce changes of the intestinal mucosa, which explains why other drugs, e.g. digitalis glycosides, may be poorly absorbed. Kuhlmann et al. [2] reported a reduced extent and rate of digoxin absorption during different combinations of cytostatic drug treatment (cyclophosphamide, vincristine, procarbazine, adriamycin, bleomycin, cytosine-arabinoside). In another study [3] it was reported that cytostatic therapy reduced the area under the plasma concentration-time curve (AUC) for verapamil by 35% after oral administration. It was concluded that the absorption of verapamil is diminished owing to impairment of the absorptive capacity of the mucosa of the upper intestine.

Methotrexate (MTX). Methotrexate given in combination with vinblastine, carmustin, and radiotherapy has been reported to decrease the plasma concentrations of phenytoin in one male patient and it was suggested that an impaired absorption of the antiepileptic drug was caused by vinblastine or methotrexate as a result of damaged small intestinal mucosa [4].

Balis et al. [5] studied the pharmacokinetics of orally administred MTX in children with acute lymphoblastic leukemia. The authors found a considerably interindividual variability in plasma levels with a bioavailability ranging from 23 to 95% (mean 62%). Their findings were later confirmed in adults [6]. The reason for the incomplete and unpredictable absorption might be a dose-dependent absorptive process for MTX, since low doses of this drug (less than 12-30 mg/m^2) were better absorbed than were higher doses [5,6]. At higher doses the absorptive carrier mechanisms are probably saturated and the bioavailability decreases [7].

In children with acute lymphocytic leukemia the bioavailability of MTX was significantly reduced by a milk meal and the authors concluded that for maximal absorption, MTX should not be taken at meal times [8]. The absorptive mechanism might not become saturated if MTX is given in divided doses and an increased absorption was also observed in children given MTX in 4 divided doses at 2-hour intervals [9].

It has also been reported that antibiotics can interfere with the absorption of MTX and with its reabsorption through enterohepatic circulation by inhibiting the bowel flora that metabolizes the drug conjugates [10].

Morphine and other related opiates have been shown to inhibit gastric emptying [11] which might delay the absorption of anticancer drugs. On the other hand, metoclopramide, which is often used to prevent nausea and vomiting in cancer patients during chemotherapy, enhances gastrointestinal motility and gastric emptying, which also may have an effect on the absorption of antineoplastic drugs [11]. Finally, the absorption characteristics of some of the anticancer drugs have been reported to be altered by food, presumably by an effect on gastric emptying. For instance, the extent of absorption of melphalan has been found to be decreased, while contradictory results have been obtained for chlorambucil [13,14]. Obviously, further studies are needed to evaluate the importance of drug-drug and food-drug interactions on the absorption of cytotoxic drugs.

Chemical Decomposition

The oral bioavailability of **melphalan** has been reported to vary between 25 and 100% [15,16]. This variability was probably related to chemical instability of melphalan in solution [17]. The chemical instability of this drug at alkaline pH was suggested as part of the mechanism behind the finding that cimetidine-induced change of gastric pH reduced the oral bioavailability of melphalan by 30% in patients with multiple myeloma [18].

Chlorambucil undergoes rapid spontaneous hydrolysis in aqueous media and an increased gastric residence time of this drug after food intake may increase the risk of hydrolysis [13].

Bioavailability and First-Pass Degradation

Bioavailability (F) is used to express the completeness of absorption and is generally

defined as the fraction of a given dose reaching the systemic circulation.
An important characteristic of drugs which show an extensive hepatic metabolism is that on oral administration the amount of drug reaching the systemic circulation may be considerably less than the dose administered (often called the first-pass effect).
As was discussed in the previous monograph on Drug Delivery in Cancer Treatment [19], the oral bioavailability (F) for a high clearance drug can be described by the following relationship:

$$F = Q / fu \times CLi \quad \text{(Eq. 1)}$$

The bioavailability is thus determined by the liver blood flow (Q), the fraction of unbound drug in plasma (fu) and the intrinsic hepatic clearance (CLi). The latter parameter expresses the total enzymatic capacity of the eliminating organ (liver) when there are no flow limitations. CLi can be determined from the ratio of dose to area under the drug concentration in blood or plasma versus time curve (AUC) after oral administration:

$$CLi = Dose_{oral} / AUC_{oral} \quad \text{(Eq. 2)}$$

The equation is valid under the assumptions that the drug is completely absorbed through the gastro-intestinal mucous membranes and is eliminated mainly by the hepatic metabolism.
On the other hand, if a high-clearance drug is given intravenously, its total plasma clearance (CL) is independent of CLi, and dependent on the liver blood flow only:

$$CL = Dose_{i.v.} / AUC_{i.v.} \approx Q \quad \text{(Eq. 3)}$$

Pharmacokinetic parameters of particular interest for the oral bioavailability of a drug with *high hepatic extraction* are thus CLi and hepatic blood flow (Q), while only the latter parameter is of interest when discussing systemic clearance after i.v. administration.

6-Mercaptopurine (6-MP). This drug has an extensive hepatic extraction with a total plasma clearance exceeding the liver plasma flow upon intravenous administration (about 1,200 ml/min/m^2 according to Zimm et al. [20]). Accordingly, one should expect a low oral bioavailability due to a prounounced first-pass degradation in the liver and possibly also in the gastrointestinal mucosa. Zimm et al. [20] showed that 4 cancer patients had an average bioavailability of 12 ± 3%.
6-MP is metabolized to 8-OH-6-MP and subsequently to inactive thiouric acid, both steps being catalyzed by xanthine oxidase [21]. Allopurinol is an inhibitor of this enzyme and the metabolic interaction between allopurinol and 6-mercaptopurin, or its imidazole precursor **azathioprine**, is one of the best known drug interactions within cancer chemotherapy [1].
In the above mentioned study [20], the authors found that the bioavailability of 6-MP increased to 59 ± 5% by pretreatment with 100 mg allopurinol three times a day for 2 days, before a 6-MP test dose of 75 mg/m^2. The maximal plasma concentration (Fig.1), the area under the plasma concentration-time curve (AUC), and bioavailability increased about 5-fold due to the same degree of decrease of intrinsic hepatic clearance (Eqs.1 and 2).
The decreased CLi being the reason for the increased bioavailability (Eq. 1) agrees with the findings of Zimm et al. [20] that the plasma concentration-time profile and the *systemic* plasma clearance (CL) of 6-MP obtained after i.v. administration were unchanged when given with or without allopurinol, since this clearance, contrary to the oral clearance (CLi), is determined only by the liver plasma flow (Eq. 3). The pharmacokinetic interaction seen between 6-MP and allopurinol is therefore most probably related to the decreased hepatic intrinsic clearance of 6-MP induced by allopurinol pretreatment and a 75% reduction of the oral dose of 6-MP is recommended when given concurrently with allopurinol [20].

In a recent paper Poplack et al. [22] raised the possibility that the low and variable oral bioavailability of 6-MP may result in subtherapeutic drug levels and might be the reason for relapses in certain patients. In addition, these authors suggested that subtherapeutic drug levels could enhance the development of drug resistance in leukemia cells. The same research group also reported that the administration of a meal (breakfast) decreased the oral AUC of 6-MP by 30% and the peak plasma concentration by about 40% [23].

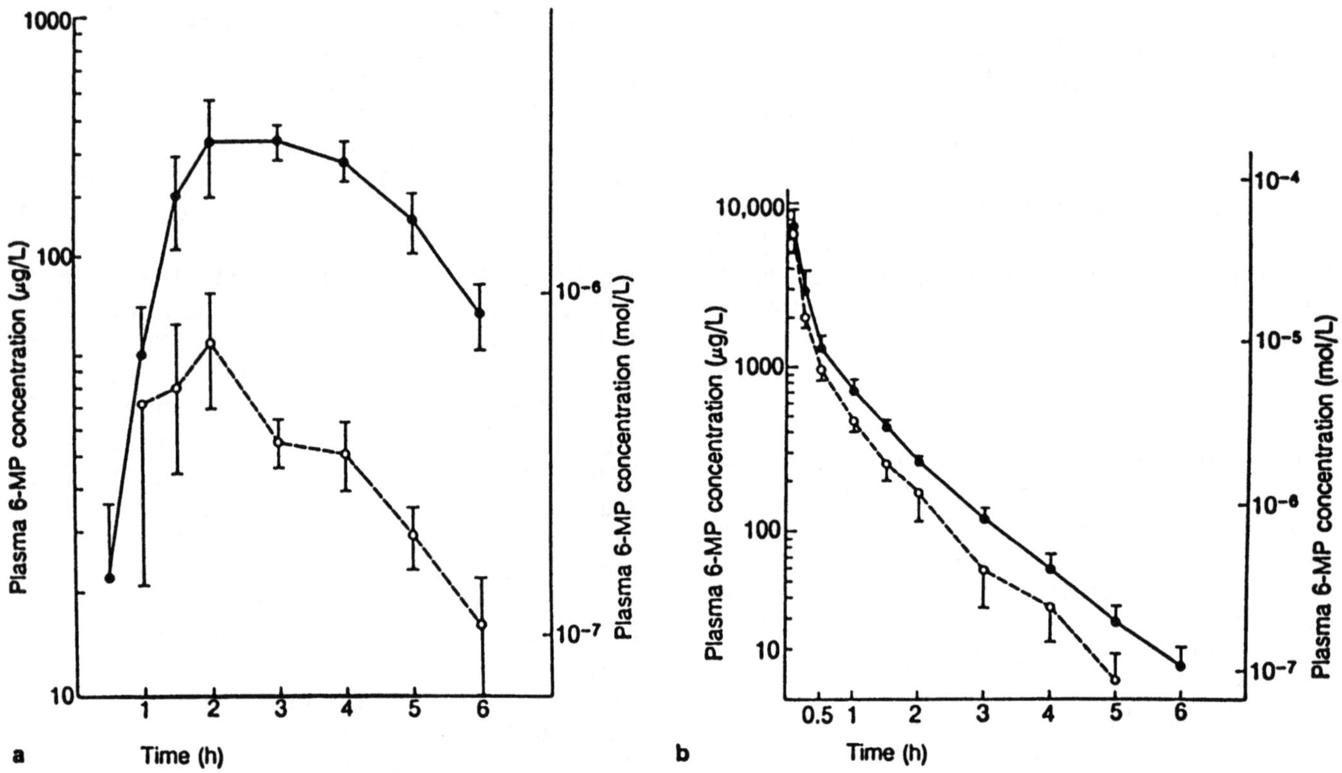

Fig. 1. Plasma concentration profiles after oral administration of 6-MP with (•) and without (o) allopurinol pretreatment (a) and following i.v. injection of 6-MP with (•) and without (o) allopurinol pretreatment (b).
Each point represents the mean ± SE from 5 patients (reproduced with permission from Zimm et al. [20])

6-Mercaptopurine is often given in combination with methotrexate and since the latter drug also has some capacity to inhibit xanthine oxidase at the level of the first-pass metabolism, it has been found that such a drug combination results in a small but significant increase in oral AUC (approx. 30%) and an increase of approx. 26% in peak plasma levels of 6-MP [24]. However, in the light of the wide interpatient variability of 6-MP bioavailability, the observed increase was not considered clinically important at standard low oral doses of methotrexate.

5-Fluorouracil (5-FU). This antimetabolic drug is mainly cleared from the body by metabolic degradation and less than 10-15% is excreted as unchanged drug in urine [25]. The hepatic plasma clearance is high and about 95% of the drug has been reported to be cleared by hepatic first-pass metabolism [26]. The bioavailability of 5-FU is consequently low and shows a high degree of interindividual variability (a range of 0-74% has been reported) [27]. Moreover, in one investigation 15% of the patients had no detectable plasma level after an oral dose of 750 mg [28]. The authors suggested a possible saturation of hepatic enzymes with increasing dose which leads to a dose-dependent bioavailability. Pretreatment with cimetidine for 4 weeks has been reported to increase peak plasma concentrations and bioavailability of 5-FU given per os [29]. There was a 27% increase of the AUC of 5-FU following i.v. administration and therefore the authors suggested that cimetidine induces a reduced hepatic blood flow (Q), thereby explaining the obtained increased bioavailability of 5-FU. However, a decreased liver blood flow will lead to a decreased bioavailability according to Eq. 1 and therefore a pronounced decrease of intrinsic hepatic clearance overcoming the potential decrease of liver blood flow is probably a more plausible ex-
The drug interactions altering absorption and discussed above are summarized in Table 1.

Table 1. Interactions altering absorption

Drug 1	Drug 2	Suggested mechanism	Effect on absorption of Drug 1
Melphalan	Cimetidine	Degradation at alkaline pH	Plasma level decreased
Azathioprin	Allopurinol	Increased bioavailability	Plasma level increased
6-Mercaptopurine	Allopurinol	Increased bioavailability	Plasma level increased
6-Mercaptopurine	Methotrexate	Increased bioavailability	Plasma level increased
Methotrexate	Antibiotics	Reduced reabsorption	Plasma level decreased
5-Fluorouracil	Cimetidine	Increased bioavailability	Plasma level increased
Digoxin	Cytostatics	Impaired absorption	Plasma level decreased
Phenytoin	Vinblastin+ Methotrexate	Impaired absorption	Plasma level decreased
Verapamil	Cytostatics	Impaired absorption	Plasma level decreased

Distribution

The apparent volume of distribution (Vd) is a primary pharmacokinetic parameter which together with the total plasma clearance (CL) determines the half-life of a drug in plasma:

$$t1/2 = 0.693 \times Vd/CL \quad \text{(Eq. 4)}$$

An increase of Vd without a concomitant change in the independent variable clearance will thus lead to a prolonged half-life [30].
A useful expression of Vd can be written as:

$$Vd = V_p + V_T \times (f_u/fu_T) \quad \text{(Eq. 5)}$$

where Vp is the physiological plasma volume (3 L) ; V_T is the volume of the extravascular space and f_u is the fraction of unbound drug in plasma. fu_T is the corresponding free fraction in tissues outside plasma [30].
From Eq. 5 it is apparent that an increased free fraction of drug in plasma (less protein-bound drug) will lead to an increased Vd, provided that tissue binding remains unchanged. (Peak concentration of a drug is affeced mainly by the size of Vd: the smaller Vd, the higher peak drug level).

Chlorambucil. A major fraction of chlorambucil is bound to serum albumin and phenylbutazone has been found to competitively displace chlorambucil from binding sites and increase the cytotoxic effect *in vitro* [31].
Methotrexate (MTX). A number of drugs have been reported to change the protein binding of MTX, mainly by displacement from serum albumin. The significance of this interaction is difficult to evaluate since a decreased protein binding (increased free fraction of drug in plasma) may according to Eq. 5 lead to increased volume of distribution. However, increase of the fraction of unbound drug may also result in an increased glomerular filtration rate and clearance (which is dependent on free drug level). Furthermore, if a renal secretion mechanism is operating, free drug levels of two or more drugs can compete for this mechanism. Thus, when considering that methotrexate has a rather low degree of plasma protein binding (50-60%) but a pronounced renal elimination, a small transient increase of free methotrexate plasma level due to displacement from albumin binding sites would normally be of little clinical significance [32]. However, patients stabilized on methotrexate who experience toxicity after being treated with a second drug should be evaluated for a drug-drug protein

interaction. Sulfonamides, salicylates, probenecid, tetracycline, chloromycetin, barbiturates, phenylbutazone, tranquilizers, and phenytoin are examples of drugs that have been reported to change the protein binding of methotrexate [1,32].

Vinca alkaloids. Vincristine and vinblastine are bound to about 75% to plasma proteins and have an extensive tissue binding leading to large volumes of distribution (8.4 L/kg and 27.3 L/kg, respectively) [33]. The large volumes are probably the main reason for the long half-lives seen for these alkaloids (Eq.4). Despite a potential risk for drug-drug protein interaction no such reports have appeared to date.

Cisplatin. This drug shows a protein binding that increases with time to more than 90% during 2-4 hours after administration [34], probably due to the formation of metabolites of cisplatin, before protein binding occurs [35]. Cisplatin accumulates in the liver and kidney where it persists for 2-4 weeks. Its clinical use is often accompanied by nephrotoxicity and a desired interaction in the kidney with other drugs in order to reduce its toxicity has been suggested. Sodium thiosulfate and acetazolamide have been investigated and according to Pfeifle et al. [36] patients tolerated about a 2-fold higher dose of cisplatin when thiosulfate was administered simultaneously.

Drug interactions altering distribution are summarized in Table 2.

Elimination

Hepatic Metabolism

After drug administration, the average plasma steady state concentration (Css) reached is determined by the ratio of the rate (amount per time) of drug administration and the total plasma clearance (CL) according to the following relationship:

$$Css = F \times Dose / Dosing\ interval \times CL \quad (Eq.\ 6)$$

Thus, besides the bioavailability (F) discussed in the previous paragraph (page 16), the plasma clearance is the only pharmacokinetic parameter that determines the actual equilibrium plasma concentration reached in the individual upon a specific dosage regimen.

Table 2. Interactions altering distribution

Drug 1	Drug 2	Suggested mechanism	Effect on Drug 1
Chlorambucil	Phenylbutazone	Displacement from plasma protein binding sites	Increased fraction of unbound drug (in vitro)
Methotrexate	Barbiturates	"	Unknown
Methotrexate	Chloromycetin	"	"
Methotrexate	Phenylbutazone	"	"
Methotrexate	Phenytoin	"	"
Methotrexate	Probenecid	"	"
Methotrexate	Salicylates	"	"
Methotrexate	Sulfonamides	"	"
Methotrexate	Tetracycline	"	"
Cisplatin	Thiosulphate	Tissue displacement?	Increased tolerability
Cisplatin	Acetazolamide	"	Unknown

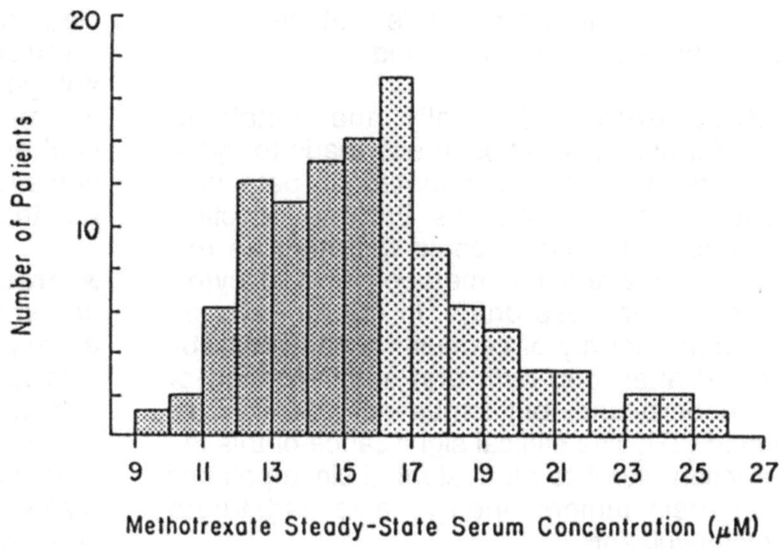

Fig. 2. Histogram of the number of patients with median steady-state serum concentrations of methotrexate in each range from a total of 108 patients receiving 1,000 mg/m^2 methotrexate, infused over 24 hrs (reproduced with permission from Evans et al. [37])

For instance, interindividual variability in methotrexate clearance among 108 children with acute lymphocytic leukemia and treated by i.v. infusion of methotrexate produced steady state serum concentrations (Fig. 2) that ranged from 9.3 to 25.4 μM [37]. Patients with median methotrexate levels less than 16 μM (n=59) had a significantly lower probability of remaining in remission than patients with concentrations of 16 μM or more. Different potential factors such as drug-drug interactions which are able to change the total plasma clearance of cytotoxic drugs might thus be of great importance for the outcome of the chemotherapy.

Cyclophosphamide. This drug produces its alkylating activity following the oxidation by hepatic microsomal enzymes (mixed-function oxidase activity). This activation produces several metabolites of varying cytotoxic potency [38], which then can be oxidized further to inactive metabolites. Drugs that can stimulate or inhibit microsomal enzymes could therefore affect the hepatic clearance of cyclophosphamide and its metabolites.

Phenobarbitone, a microsomal enzyme inducer, could consequently be expected to increase the rate of metabolism of cyclophosphamide and this has been observed in a number of animal studies [1]. However, the clinical importance of this finding is unclear, since most studies have been performed in animals. Jao et al. [39] found that phenobarbitone increased the biotransformation of cyclophosphamide 2- to 3-fold, but it did not change the total amount of alkylating metabolites. These authors therefore concluded that the therapeutic effect of cyclophosphamide remains relatively unchanged following phenobaritone pretreatment. Further studies are obviously needed in this matter.

Cyclophosphamide can also induce its own metabolism during repeated dosing. Decreased half-life of cyclophosphamide during treatment has been observed [40-42] as well as increased plasma levels of alkylating metabolites [43]. However, with low doses, no change in the pharmacokinetics of cyclophosphamide was found [44].

Cimetidine, a well-known inhibitor of oxidative hepatic enzymes, has been reported by Dorr and Alberts [45] to increase the plasma concentrations of alkylating metabolites of cyclophosphamide in mice, but this interaction has not been studied in man. The authors, however, pointed out that caution should be observed when using cimetidine in combina-

tion with full doses of cyclophosphamide or other anticancer drugs metabolized by microsomal enzymes.
Further studies of the kinetics of especially the metabolites are obviously needed before the clinical importance of enzyme induction or inhibition of cyclophosphamide metabolism by other drugs can be determined

Nitrosoureas. Generally, the metabolic transformation of nitrosoureas leads to cytotoxic products and the metabolic pathways include hepatic oxidations. Enzyme induction after phenobarbitone could therefore be expected to affect the metabolism and cytotoxicity after these drugs. In the rat, reduced antitumor activity of carmustine has been observed after long-term oral administration of phenobarbitone, but lomustine was less affected [27]. The clinical significance of this interaction ought to be evaluated since patients with brain tumors often receive barbiturate anticonvulsants.

6-Mercaptopurine and Azathioprine. Allopurinol inhibits competitively xanthine oxidase and consequently the metabolism of 6-MP. This type of interaction is, as mentioned before (page 17), of importance only when 6-mercaptopurine is given orally but not by the i.v. route. However, allopurinol can inhibit the renal secretion of unchanged 6-MP and its metabolite thiouric acid (page 23), which could lead to a potential toxicity [20]. As mentioned before (page 17), also methotrexate inhibits xanthine oxidase, which metabolizes 6-mercaptopurine, and the consequences of this interaction were discussed in connection with the absorption characteristics of 6-MP.

5-Fluorouracil. 5-FU exhibits a high hepatic clearance but also a dose-dependent metabolism probably by saturation of catabolic enzymes at higher doses [46]. Thymidine or thymine (the metabolite of thymidine) reduces the total plasma clearance of 5-FU as a result of a competitive inhibition of dihydrouracil dehydrogenase by circulating thymine [47]. The total clearance of 5-FU was shown to be reduced from 18.9 L/min to 2.7 L/min by a concurrent 5-day infusion of thymidine in man, yielding thymidine concentrations of 20-30 μmol/L.
As mentioned in relation to the absorption characteristics of 5-FU, cimetidine given for 4 weeks before an oral dose of 5-FU decreases the intrinsic hepatic clearance of 5-FU. Misonidazole, with a chemical structure similar to cimetidine, is also able to reduce the clearance of 5-FU in humans [48].
Methotrexate has been reported to antagonize or potentiate the effects of 5-FU via an inhibition of thymidylate synthetase. Higher concentrations of methotrexate, however, can increase the enzyme activity and thus overcome its antagonistic effect [49].

Antracyclines. The antracyclines are excreted mainly by the hepatobiliary system with a hepatic extraction ratio of 0.5-0.6. Cyclophosphamide is often used concurrent with adriamycin; the former drug, however, can alter the metabolism of the latter. The plasma concentrations of adriamycin remained unchanged in children when used in combination with cyclophosphamide, but the further metabolism of its active alcohol, adriamycinol, to aglycones was inhibited since increased serum concentration of the alcohol was observed [52].
The drug interactions altering hepatic metabolism and discussed above are summarized in Table 3.

Renal Elimination

Cyclophosphamide. About 6.5-20% of the given dose of cyclophosphamide is excreted unchanged in the urine [51]. The excretion of active metabolites is decreased in patients with renal function impairment (creatinine clearance < 20 ml/min) and a dose reduction is recommended only in patients with severe renal dysfuntion [52,53]. It has been reported that allopurinol increases the metabolite plasma AUC of cyclophosphamide, but the mechanism of this interaction is unclear and may be due to a decrease in the renal clearance of metabolites caused by allopurinol [54]. Allopurinol has also been reported to increase the myelotoxicity induced by cyclophosphamide when the drugs were given concurrently [27].

Table 3. Interactions altering hepatic metabolism

Drug 1	Drug 2	Suggested mechanism	Effect on Drug 1
Cyclophosphamide	Cyclophosphamide	Induction of enzymes	Decreased half-life Increase of alkylating metabolites in plasma
Cyclophosphamide (animals)	Cimetidine	Inhibition of enzymes	Increase of alkylating metabolites in plasma
Nitrosoureas (animals)	Phenobarbitone	Induction of enzymes	Reduced antitumor activity
6-Mercaptopurine	Methotrexate	Inhibition of enzymes	Increased plasma levels
6-Mercaptopurine	Allopurinol (only per os)	Inhibition of enzymes	Increased plasma levels
5-Fluorouracil	Thymine, Thymidine	Inhibition of enzymes	" " "
5-Fluorouracil	Cimetidine	Plasma clearance decreased	" " "
5-Fluorouracil	Misonidazole	" " "	" " "
Adriamycin	Cyclophosphamide	Inhibition of enzymes	Increased plasma levels of adriamycinol

6-Mercaptopurine. Allopurinol administered during 6-MP infusion caused a 60% reduction of the urinary excretion of the metabolite thiouric acid and about 20% increase of the excretion of unchanged 6-MP in relation to the administered dose. A potential risk of unexpected toxicity in patients with renal dysfunction given concurrent allopurinol and 6-MP was therefore suggested [20].

Methotrexate. Plasma clearance of methotrexate is in man about 108 ml/min and the renal clearance is about 104 ml/min. Administered with probenecid these figures were reduced to 69 ml/min and 46 ml/min, respectively [55]. The decreased plasma clearance leads to increased plasma levels of methotrexate [56].

Like probenecid other organic acids will compete with methotrexate for the renal tubular transport system. Thus, salicylates, sulfafurazole, phenylbutazone, and penicillin are examples of such competition with methotrexate [1,32,57,58]. Salicylates have been shown to decrease the renal clearance of low-dose methotrexate by up to 35% [57]. Concomitant use of salicylates and methotrexate has been found to increase the incidence of toxicity [59].

Ketoprofen and indomethacin, two nonsteroidal antiinflammatory agents, have been reported to cause fatal toxicity when used together with methotrexate [60,61]. The simultaneous administration of high-dose methotrexate and ketoprofen was associated with prolonged and striking enhancement of serum methotrexate plasma levels. There were, however, no changes in methotrexate pharmacokinetics or toxicity when ketoprofen was given at least 12 hours after the high-dose methotrexate infusion [60]. The explanation to this interaction is not very straightforward. Thyss and associates [60] suspected a defect in the clearance of methotrexate as being the mechanism of this interaction and they suggested that the inhibition of the prostaglandin synthesis by ketoprofen might decrease the renal perfusion and consequently methotrexate clearance. An alternative could be the competition of the two drugs for the renal tubular transport system, as discussed above. Thyss et al. [60] also warned that a severe interaction might be anticipated for other NSAIDs since these drugs are often used in the management of pain in cancer patients.

Maiche [62] reported one case of acute renal failure due to concomitant use of methotrexate and indomethacin. He also suggested that this interaction could be due to a decrease of the renal clearance of methotrexate but did not exclude other possibilities of an interaction at the biotransformation steps. A report of a lethal interaction between naproxen and an overdose of methotrexate has also recently appeared [63]. Other NSAIDs that have been reported to cause toxic interactions with methotrexate are azapropazone [64] and diclofenac [60].

An alternative explanation for the interaction between NSAIDs and methotrexate could be a displacement of methotrexate from plasma proteins [65,66]. However, methotrexate is bound to plasma proteins only to about 50% [67]. If a displacement were of clinical significance, the displaced compound would be bound to about 90% or more and it would have a small volume of distribution [68]. Since methotrexate has a rather moderate volume of distribution (about 1 L/kg), the displacement phenomenon is not a likely explanation for the above discussed interactions. Slordal et al. [69] have, however, suggested that a displacement of the major metabolite of methotrexate, 7-hydroxy-methotrexate, bound to about 90-93% and with a volume of distribution much less than methotrexate, could be the reason for the serious interaction between NSAIDs and methotrexate. This metabolite is cytotoxic *in vitro* and has been suggested to be responsible for renal toxicity [70]. Slordal and associates [69] have also shown that the serum concentration of this metabolite increases 2- to 3-fold in volunteers after administration of 1000 mg naproxen.

Drugs that impair renal function should be able to change the clearance of methotrexate. The nephrotoxic effect of cisplatin has been suggested to be the cause of the interaction between this drug and methotrexate [71,72]. Crom et al. [71] suggested that a delayed clearance is likely to be found in children with a total dose of 360 mg/m^2 or more of cisplatin and these authors recommended that this high-risk group of patients could benefit from using a test dose of methotrexate to reveal their plasma clearance prior to the use of high doses of methotrexate.

Other potentially nephrotoxic drugs such as aminoglycosides and amphotericin B also have the potential to decrease the renal elimination of methotrexate [73,74].

Bleomycin. This drug is mainly eliminated by renal excretion and severe toxicity has been observed in patients with renal dysfunction [75,76]. Cisplatin with its nephrotoxic potential has been reported to decrease the total clearance of bleomycin when the cumulative dose of cisplatin exceeded 300 mg/m^2 [77].

Cisplatin. Cisplatin is eliminated mainly by the kidneys [34]. Since the protein binding increases over time to more than 90%, the renal clearance will likewise decrease over time and result in a prolonged excretory phase and only 27-45% of the dose is excreted over 3.5-5 days [34,78]. Besides glomerular filtration cisplatin is also secreted by the renal tubules. Consequently, probenecid pretreatment significantly reduces the renal clearance of filterable platinum [79].

The drug interactions altering renal elimination and discussed above are summarized in Table 4.

Drug-Plastic Interactions

Today, mixtures or single-drug preparations of anticancer drugs are routinely administered by continuous i.v. infusions during a relatively long period of time. Alternatively the drugs may be delivered loco-regionally for a prolonged period. New technical devices are frequently introduced in the field of cancer chemotherapy to facilitate and optimize drug treatment in patients. Simultaneously, schedules for drug administration have been carefully elaborated to improve the accuracy of drug dosing.

It is, however, of great importance to coordinate the different components included in the development of new strategies for administration of anticancer drugs. There seems to be a gap between manufacturers responsible for administration systems and manufacturers responsible for the drug products, in that very sparse information about drug-plastic, drug-glass and drug-inline filter material interactions is available.

Table 4. Interactions altering renal elimination

Drug 1	Drug 2	Suggested mechanism	Effect on Drug 1
Cyclophosphamide	Allopurinol	Decrease in renal clearance	Increased plasma metabolites
6-Mercaptopurine	Allopurinol	Unclear	Increased excretion of unchanged drug; decreased excretion of metabolites
Methotrexate	Probenecid	Decrease in renal clearance	Increased plasma levels
Methotrexate	Salicylates	Decrease in renal clearance	Increased toxicity
Methotrexate	Sulphafurazole	Decrease in renal clearance	Unknown
Methotrexate	Phenylbutazone	Decrease in renal clearance	Unknown
Methotrexate	Penicillin	Decrease in renal clearance	Unknown
Methotrexate	Ketoprofen	Unclear	Increased plasma levels and toxicity
Methotrexate	Indomethacin	Unclear	Renal impairment
Methotrexate	Naproxen	Unclear	Increased toxicity (lethal)
Methotrexate	Azapropazone	Unclear	Increased toxicity
Methotrexate	Diclophenac	Unclear	Increased toxicity
Methotrexate	Cisplatin	Nephrotoxicity	Increased half-life and toxicity
Methotrexate	Aminoglycosides	Nephrotoxicity	Decreased renal elimination?
Methotrexate	Amphotericin B	Nephrotoxicity	" "
Bleomycin	Cisplatin	Nephrotoxicity	Plasma clearance decreased
Cisplatin	Probenecid	Renal clearance decreased	Unknown

Undoubtedly, interactions between plastic material and antineoplastic substances should not be neglected. For example, the sorption of carmustine in common standard administration sets of polyvinylchloride (PVC) from 5 different manufacturers were examined by Fredriksson et al. [80]. All sets showed a similar high sorption of carmustin; after 5 minutes' exposure the drug loss was 10% and after 2 hours only 35% of the drug was left in the stationary solution (0.01 M citrate buffer, pH 4.2). Different sets made of different plastic polymers were tested and in both polyurethane and ethylenevinyl acetate copolymer (EVA) there was a considerable loss of drug (for polyurethane less than 20% of the drug was left in the stationary solution after 2 hours). However, a combination set made of polyethylene internally and EVA externally was almost resistant to sorption [80]. The above-mentioned authors also investigated the variation of carmustine concentration during drug infusion using PVC infusion sets at different flow rates. After 1 hour of infusion with a flow rate of 530 ml/h, 4.6 % of the dose was lost. With a flow rate of 530 ml/2h the loss was 8.1% after the first hour and with a flow rate of 530 ml/6h the loss increased to 23% of the amount of carmustine passed during the first hour. In the above experiments light, temperature, and pH were chosen so as to keep maximal stability of carmustine. In the flow rate experiments, isotonic dextrose in a glass bottle was used as infusion fluid.

Benvenuto et al. [81] determined the stability of a number of anticancer drugs in underfilled polyvinyl chloride bags and glass bottles. The drugs were reconstituted according to the manufacturers' instructions. All admixtures were stored at room temperature, not protected from light. For the majority of antitumor drugs, no significant differences between the stability in plastic vs. glass containers were found; however, there were a number of exceptions. Fluorouracil and doxorubicin were more stable in plastic than in glass containers, whereas bleomycin sulfate and carmustine were stable only in glass containers. Mitomycin was not stable in either glass or plastic. Later, Biondi and Nairn [82] showed that 5-fluorouracil at therapeutic concentrations was very stable in both plastic bags and glass bottle containers, provided that the solution was kept in filled containers.

Inline i.v. filters containing a cellulose ester membrane have been found to bind dactinomycin [83] and vincristine sulfate [84] resulting in substantial loss of drug amount. When the filter membrane was pretreated with an agent minimizing the binding, untreated filters bound 5-7 times as much of vincristine sulfate and dactinomycin as did the treated filter in equilibrium binding studies [85].

A review of the available documentation on drug-plastic and drug-glass interactions of anticancer agents shows that not only is the information scanty, when it exists at all, it is often incomplete. The literature lacks broad investigations where attention has been paid to the importance of standardized experimental conditions. This lack of basic information is surprising and, of course, not acceptable. It is obvious that a number of factors affect the results and the conclusions drawn in one investigation might be erroneous under different experimental circumstances. It is therefore mandatory to design investigations in such a way as to reflect the clinical situation in which the drug is administered to the patient.

REFERENCES

1 Balis FM: Pharmacokinetic drug interactions of commonly used anticancer drugs. Clin Pharmacokin 1986 (11):223-235

2 Kuhlmann J, Zilly W and Wilke J: Effects of cytostatic drugs on plasma level and renal excretion of ß-acetyldigoxin. Clin Pharmacol Ther 1981 (30):518-527

3 Kuhlman J, Woodcock B, Wilke J and Rietbrock N: Verapamil plasma concentrations during treatment with cytostatic drugs. J Cardiovasc Pharmacol 1985 (7):1003-1006

4 Bollini P, Riva R, Albani F, Ida N, Cacciari L, Bollini C and Baruzzi A: Decreased Phenytoin level during antineoplastic therapy: a case report. Epilepsia 1983 (24):75-78

5 Balis FM, Savitch JL and Bleyer WA: The pharmacokinetics of oral methotrexate in children. Cancer Res 1983 (43):23-45

6 Campbell MA, Perrier DG, Dorr RT, Alberts DS and Finley PR: Methotrexate: Bioavailability and pharmacokinetics. Cancer Treat Rep 1985 (69):833-838

7 Smith DK, Omura GA and Ostroy F: Clinical pharmacology of intermediate - dose oral methotrexate. Cancer Chemother Pharmacol 1980 (4):117-120

8 Pinkerton CR, Glasgow JFT, Welshman SG and Bridges JM: Can food influence the absorption of methotrexate in children with acute lymphoblastic leukemia? Lancet 1980 (2):944-946

9 Steel WH, Stuart JFB and Lawrence JR: Enhancement of methotrexate absorption by subdivision of dose. Cancer chemother Pharmacol 1979 (3):235-237

10 Shen DD and Azarnoff D: Clinical pharmacokinetics of methotrexate. Clin Pharmacokin 1978 (3):1-13

11 Jaffe JH and Martin WR: Opoid analgesics and antagonists. In: Gilman AG, Goodman LS, Rall TW and Murad F (eds) The pharmacological basis of therapeutics. Macmillan Publishing Company New York, 1985 p 502

12 Gralla RJ, Itri LM, Pisko SE, Squillante AE and Kelsen DP: Antiemetic efficacy of high dose metoclopramide randomized trials with placebo and prochlorperazine in patients with chemotherapy-induced nausea and vomiting. New Engl J Med 1981 (305):905-909

13 Adair CG, Bridges JM and Desai ZR: Can food affect the bioavailability of chlorambucil in patients with haematological malignancies? Cancer Chemother Pharmacol 1986 (17):99-102

14 Ehrsson H, Wallin I, Simonsson B, Hartvig P and Öberg G: Effect of food on the pharmacokinetics of chlorambucil and its main metabolite, phenylacetic acid mustard. Eur J Clin Pharmacol 1984 (27):111

15 Alberts DS, Chang SY, Chen HS, Evans TL and Moon TE: Oral melphalan kinetics: Clin Pharmacol Ther 1979 (26):737-745

16 Woodhouse KW, Hamilton P, Lennard A and Rawlins MD: The pharmacokinetics of melphalan in patients with multiple myeloma. Eur J Clin Pharmacol 1983 (24):283-285

17 Bosanquet AG: Stability of melphalan solutions during preparation and storage. J Pharm Sci 1985 (74):348-351

18 Sviland L, Robinson A, Proctor SJ and Bateman DN: Interaction of cimetidine with oral melphalan. A pharmacokinetic study. Cancer Chemother Pharmacol 1987 (20):173-175

19 Paalzow LK: How physiological and pathophysiological factors influence the pharmacokinetics and analgesic effect of opiates in cancer patients. In: Domellöf L (ed) Drug delivery in cancer treatment. Springer-Verlag Berlin Heidelberg 1987 pp 19-27

20 Zimm S, Collins JM, O'Neill D, Chabner BA and Poplack DG: Inhibition of first-pass metabolism in cancer chemotherapy: Interaction of 6-mercaptopurine and allopurinol. Clin Pharmacol Ther 1983 (34): 810-817

21 Elion GB: Biochemistry and pharmacology of purine analogues. Fed Proc 1967 (26):898-904

22 Poplack DG, Balis FM and Zimm S: The pharmacology of orally administered chemotherapy. Cancer 1986 (Suppl July 15):473-480

23 Riccardi R, Balis F, Ferrara P, Lasorella A, Poplack D and Mastrangelo R: Influence of food intake on the absorption of orally administered 6-mercaptopurine (6-MP). Proc Am Soc Clin Oncol 1985 (4):34

24 Balis FM, Holcenberg JS, Zimm S, Tubergen D, Collins JM, Murphy RF, Gilchrist GS, Hammond D and Poplack DG: The effect of methotrexate on the bioavailability of oral 6-mercaptopurine. Clin Pharmacol Ther 1987 (41):384-387

25 Sitar DS, Shaw DH, Thirwell MP and Rendy JR: Disposition of 5-fluorouracil after intravenous bolus doses of a commerical formulation to cancer patients. Cancer Res 1977 (37):3981-3984

26 Finn C and Sadee W: Determination of 5-fluorouracil (NSC-19893) plasma levels in rats and man by isotope dilution-mass fragmentography. Cancer Chemother Rep 1975 (59):279-286

27 Balis FM, Holcenberg JS and Bleyer WA: Clinical pharmacokinetics of commonly used anticancer drugs. Clin Pharmacokin 1983 (8):202-232

28 Christophidis N, Vajda FJE, Lucus J, Drummer O,Moon WJ and Louis WJ: Fluorouracil therapy in patients with carcinoma of the large bowel: a pharmacokinetic comparison of various rates and routes of administration. Clin Pharmacokin 1978 (3):330-336

29 Harvey VJ, Slevin ML, Dilloway MR, Clark PJ and Johnston A: The influence of cimetidine on the pharmacokinetics of 5-fluorouracil. Brit J Clin Pharmacol 1984 (18):421-430

30 Rowland M and Tozer TN: Distribution. In: Clinical Pharmacokinetics: concepts and applications. Lea & Febiger, Philadelphia 1980 pp 34-47

31 Schiffman FJ, Uehara Y, Fisher JM and Rabinovitz M: Potentiation of chlorambucil activity by phenylbutazone. Cancer Letters 1978 (4):211-216

32 Evans WE and Christensen ML: Drug interactions with methotrexate. J Rheumatol 1985 (suppl 12)12):15-20

33 Nelson RL, Dyke RW and Root MA: Comparative pharmacokinetics of vindesine, vincristine and

vinblastine in patients with cancer. Cancer Treatm Rev 7 1980 (suppl):17-24
34 DeConti RC, Toftness BR, Lange RC and Creasy WA: Clinical and pharmacological studies with cisdiamminedichloroplatinum II. Cancer Res 1973 (33):1310-1315
35 LeRoy AF, Lutz RJ, Dedrik RL, Litterst CL and Guarino AM: Pharmacokinetic study of cis-dichlorodiammineplatinum (II)(DDP) in the beagle dog: thermodynamic and kinetic behaviour of DDP in a biologic milieu. Cancer Treatm Rep 1979 (63):59-71
36 Pfeifle CF, Howell SB, Felthouse RD, Woliver TBS and Andrews PA: High dose cisplatin with sodium thiosulphate protection. J Clin Oncol 1985 (3):237-244
37 Evans WE, Crom WR, Abromovitch M, Dodge R, Look AT, Bowman WP, George SL and Pui CH: Clinical pharmacodynamics of high-dose methotrexate in acute lymphocytic leukemia. New Eng J Med 1986 (314):471-477
38 Grochow LB and Colvin M: Clinical pharmacokinetics of cyclophosphamide. Clin Pharmacokin 1979 (4):380-394
39 Fao JY, Fusko WJ and Cohen JL: Phenobarbital effects on cyclophosphamide pharmacokinetics in man. Cancer Res 1972 (32):2761-2764
40 D'Incalci M, Bolis G, Facchinetti T, Mangioni C and Morasca L: Decreased half life of cyclophosphamide in patients under continual treatment. Europ J Cancer 1979 (15):7-10
41 Graham MI, Shaw IC, Souhami RL, Sidau B and Harper PG: Decreased plasma half-life of cyclophosphamide during repeated high-dose administration. Cancer Chemother and Pharmacol 1983 (10):192-193
42 Sladck NE, Priest J, Doeden D, Mirocha CJ and Pathre S: Plasma half-life and urinary excretion of cyclophosphamide in children. Cancer Treatm Rep 1980 (64):1061-1066
43 Bagley CM, Bostich FW and De Vita VT: Clinical pharmacology of cyclophosphamide. Cancer Res 1973 (33):226-233
44 Mouridsen HT, Faber O and Skovsted L: The metabolism of cyclophosphamide. Cancer 1976 (37):665-670
45 Dorr DI and Alberts DS: Cimetidine enhancement of cyclophosphamide antitumor activity. Br J Cancer 1982 (45):35-43
46 Collins JM, Dedrik RL, King FG, Speyer JL and Myers CE: Nonlinear pharmacokinetic models for 5-flurouracil in man: intravenous and intraperitoneal routes. Clin Pharmacol Ther 1980 (28):235-246
47 Au JL-S, Rustum YM, Ledesma EJ, Mittelman A and Creaven PJ: Clinical pharmacological studies of concurrent infusion of 5-fluorouracil and thymidine in treatment of colorectal carcinomas. Cancer Res 1982 (42):2930-2937
48 Mc Dermott BJ, Van der Berg HW, Martin WMC and Murphy RF: Pharmacokinetic rationale for the interaction of 5-fluorouracil and misonidazole in humans. Br J Cancer 1983 (48):705-710
49 Bertino JR: Toward improved selectivity in cancer chemotherapy. Cancer Res 1979 (39):293-304
50 Evans WE, Crom WR, Sinjule JA, Yee GC and Stewart CF: Pharmacokinetics of anticancer drugs in children. Drug Metabol Rew 1983 (14): 847-886
51 Juma FD, Rogers HJ and Trounce JR: Pharmacokinetics of cyclophosphamide and alkylating activity in man after intravenous and oral administration. Br J Clin Pharmacol 1979 (8):209-217
52 Mouridsen HT and Jacobsen E: Pharmacokinetics of cyclophosphamide in renal failure. Acta Pharmacol et Tox 1975 (36):409-414
53 Bagley CM, Bostich FW and De Vita VT: Clinical pharmacology of cyclophosphamide. Cancer Res 1973 (33):226-233
54 Witten S, Frederiksen PL and Mouridsen HT: The pharmacokinetics of cyclophosphamide in man after treatment with allopurinol. Acta Pharmacol et Tox 1980 (46):392-394
55 Aherne GW, Piall E, Marks V, Mould G and White WF: Prolongation and enhancement of serum methotrexate concentrations by probenecid. Br Med J 1978 (1):1097-1099
56 Howell SB, Olshen RA and Rice JA: Effect of probenecid on cerebrospinal fluid methotrexate kinetics. Clin Pharmacol Ther 1979 (26): 641-646
57 Liegler DG, Henderson ES, Hahn MA and Oliverio VT: The effect of organic acids on renal clearance of methotrexate in man. Clin Pharmacol Ther 1969 (10):849-857
58 Williams WM, Chen TS and Huang KC: Effect of pencillin on the renal tubular secretion of methotrexate in the monkey. Cancer Res 1984 (44):1913-1917
59 Mandel MA: The synergistic effect of salicylates on methotrexate toxicity. Plastic and Reconstructive Surg 1976 (57):733-739
60 Thyss A, Milano G, Kubar J, Namer M and Schneider M: Clinical and pharmacokinetic evidence of a life treatening interaction between methotrexate and ketoprofen. Lancet 1986 (1):256-258
61 Ellison NM and Servi RJ: Acute renal failure and death following sequential intermediate-dose methotrexate and 5-FU: a possible adverse effect due to concomitant indomethacin administration. Cancer Treatm Rep 1985 (69):342-343
62 Maiche AG: Acute renal failure due to concomitant action of methotrexate and indomethacin. Lancet 1986 (1):1390
63 Singh RR, Malaviya AN, Pandey JN and Guleria JS: Fatal interaction between methotrexate and naproxen. Lancet 1986 (1):1390
64 Daly H, Boyle J, Roberts C and Scott G: Interaction between methotrexate and non-steroidal anti-inflammatory drugs. Lancet 1986 (1): 557
65 Ng HWK, MacFarlane AW, Graham RM and Verbov JL: Near fatal drug interactions with methotrexate given for psoriasis. Br Med J 1987 (295):752-753
66 Thomas MH and Gutterman LA: Methotrexate toxicity in a patient receiving trimethoprim-sulphamethoxazole. J Reumatol 1986 (13): 440-441
67 Paxton JW: The protein binding and elimination of methotrexate after intravenous infusions in cancer patients. Clin Exp Pharmacol Physiol 1982 (9):225-234

68 Dettli L: Pharmacokinetic aspects of drug interactions. In: Cluff LE and Petric JC (eds) Clinical effects of interaction between drugs. Elsevier, New York 1974 pp 39-68
69 Slordal L, Sager G and Aarbakke J: Pharmacokinetic interactions with methotrexate: is 7-hydroxy-methotrexate the culprit? Lancet1988 (1):591-592
70 Jacobs SA, Stoller RG, Chabner BA and Johns DG: 7-Hydroxy-methotrexate as a urinary metabolite in human subjects and rhesus monkeys receiving high-dose methotrexate. J Clin Invest 1976 (57):534-538
71 Crom WR, Pratt CB, Green AA, Campion JE and Crom DB: The effects of prior cisplatin therapy on the pharmacokinetics of high-dose methotrexate. J Clin Oncol 1984 (2):655-661
72 Haim N, Kedar A and Robinson E: Methotrexate-related deaths in patients previously treated with cis-diammine dichloride platinum. Cancer Chem and Pharmacol 1984 (13):223-225
73 Schentag JJ, Plant ME and Cerra FB: Aminoglycoside nephrotoxicity in critically ill surgical patients. J Surg Res 1979 (26):270-279
74 Smith CR, Maxwell RR and Edward CQ: Nephrotoxicity induced by gentamicin and amikacin. John Hopkins Med J 1978 (142):85-90
75 Bennett WM, Pastore L and Houghton DC: Fatal pulmonary toxicity in cisplatin-induced acute renal failure. Cancer Treatm Rep 1980 (64): 921-924
76 Perry DJ, Weiss RB and Taylor HG: Enhanced bleomycin toxicity during acute renal failure. Cancer Treatm Rep 1982 (66):592-593
77 Yee GC, Crom WR, Campion JE, Brodeur GM and Evans WE: Cisplatin-induced changes in bleomycin elimination. Cancer Treatm Rep 1983 (67):587-589
78 Smith PHS and Taylor DM: Distribution and retention of the antitumor agent 195m-Pt-cis-dichlorodiammine platinum (II) in man. J Nucl Med 1974 (15):349-351
79 Jacobs C, Coleman CN, Rich L, Hirst K and Weiner MW: Inhibition of cis-diamminedichloroplatinum secretion by the human kidney with probenecid. Cancer Res 1984 (44):3632-3635
80 Fredriksson K, Lundgren P and Landersjö L: Stability of carmustine kinetics and compatibility during administration. Acta Pharm Suec 1986 (23):115-124
81 Benvenuto JA, Andersson RW, Kerhof K, Smith RG and Loo TL: Stability and compatibility of antitumor agents in glass and plastic containers. Am J Hosp Pharm 1981 (38):1914-1918
82 Biondi L and Nairn JG: Stability of 5-Fluorouracil and flucytosine in parenteral solutions. The Can J Hosp Pharm 1986 (39):60-64
83 De Luca PP: Binding of drugs to inline filters. Am J Hosp Pharm 1979 (36):151-154
84 Butler LD, Munson JM and De Luca PP: Effect of inline filtration on the potency of low-dose drugs. Am J Hosp Pharm 1980 (37):935-941
85 Kanke M, Eubanks JL and De Luca PP: Binding of selected drugs to a "treated" inline filter. Am J Hosp Pharm 1983 (40):1323-1328

Immunotherapy and Interactions of Cytokines in the Host

K.G. Lundholm

Department of Surgery, Sahlgrenska Hospital, University of Gothenburg, Sweden

Introduction

A successful outcome from any form of cancer treatment must depend on those features of a tumor which make it distinct in some way from the surrounding normal tissue. In surgery and radiation therapy this aspect is fulfilled by the histological and gross anatomical delineation of tumor tissue. Chemotherapy and immunotherapy are rather dependent on specific or unique features in metabolism, microstructures and on the molecular appearance of tumor cells compared to normal untransformed tissues. However, the lack of adequacy in controlling most malignant tumors demonstrates our present incapacity to define and apply this strategy. Nevertheless, modern medicine and hopefully also cancer treatment will benefit from the rapid development of molecular biology. The purpose of this presentation is to summarize briefly old and recent concepts of immune-interventions in cancer patients and discuss some aspects of a continuously expanding research field of cytokines and growth factors in a way that may have a bearing on the clinical horizon. Cytokines include both monokines and lymphokines, the latter referring to the cellular origin of synthesis, i.e., monocytes and lymphocytes.

Specific Passive Immunotherapy

As early as 1895 Hericourt and Richet published a brief note on serotherapy in the treatment of cancer [1]. Since then hundreds of patients have been evaluated following infusion of antisera from both animals and patients immunized with tumor tissue and antigens from various sources [2]. So far, passive immunization has not provided any real basis for optimism concerning the clinical value of this approach.

Non-Specific Active Immunotherapy

Non-specific boosting of immunological reactivity has been used in many forms in treatment of both animals and humans. The immune response to a variety of antigens from yeasts, mycobacteria, tubercle bacteria (BCG), zymosan, shark liver lipids, polysaccharides extracted from bagasse, wheatstraw, bamboo leaves, edible mushrooms, Proteus vulgaris and Corynebacterium parvum have been used. There is, however, little evidence that such agents have any therapeutic effect either in man or in animals. Most test systems of non-specific immune stimulation involve pretreatment of the host before the tumor challenge in order to be effective. Indeed, it has even been suggested that non-specific immunization may enhance tumor growth when given alone to tumor-bearing animals.

Adoptive Immunotherapy

Adoptive immunotherapy of cancer can be defined as the transfer to the tumor-bearing host of lymphoid cells with antitumor reactivity that can mediate directly or indirectly the regression of the tumor. The use of immune cells in cancer treatment is a relatively recent development. It is based on the demonstration of the powerful effect of these cell types in transplantation immunity. Immune reactions to tumor or tumor-associated antigens, which are an integrated part of the cell membrane, are usually of the delayed hypersensitivity type. This form of reaction can be adoptively transferred from one individual to another with lymphoid cells.

One initial and large series of patients treated with adoptive immunotherapy was that described by Nadler and Moore [3]. They cross-immunized pairs of patients with their respective tumors and subsequently exchanged sensitized peripheral blood lymphocytes. This design is, however, subject to severe conceptual criticism. Induction of immunity to transplantation antigens (HLA) would rapidly destroy the transfused lymphoid cells. No convincing curative treatment effect was reported, although some improvement of well-being was suggested.

A similar approach in a smaller group of patients has been reported using thoracic duct lymphocytes from patients "immunized" with tumor [4]. Using this technique, the authors were able to transfer large amounts of lymphoid cells. No objective response was observed in treatment of patients with leukemia and melanoma and graft-versus-host reactions may have supervened.

Trouillas and Lapras [5] have employed autologous lymphocytes from patients "autoimmunized" against their own cerebral tumors. Thoracic duct lymphocytes were isolated and injected into the cerebral fluid in an attempt to bypass the blood-brain barrier. No clinical benefit was achieved but post-mortem examinations of tumor specimens revealed significant immune-cell infiltration; this was probably a random finding.

Modern Approaches to Immunotherapy

Based on the examples given above it is obvious that more refined and specific approaches must be adopted in order to be able to control cancer growth. In this effort it is anticipated that specificity must be combined with convenience if one wishes to apply a regimen on a large-scale treatment basis in average hospitals.

Adoptive immunotherapy with transfer to the tumor-bearing host of cells with antitumor reactivity is an attractive approach. This concept in its modern fashion is based on the observation that the incubation of murine and human lymphocytes in the presence of the lymphokine interleukin-2 (IL-2), led to the generation of cells with the ability to lyse fresh non-cultured tumor cells [6,7]. More recent results have shown that this effect should be ascribed to generation and activation of lymphokine-activated killer (LAK) cells [8,9]. These cells are capable of lysing natural killer-resistant (NK) tumor cells but not normal untransformed cells. LAK cells can be produced by incubating samples of peripheral blood lymphocytes with high concentrations of IL-2 for 2-3 days. This procedure induces the activation of a cell type (LAK) that is distinct from both natural killer cells and cytolytic T-lymphocytes [10]. LAK precursor cells do not express T-cell markers, although the LAK effector cells express classic T cell markers. Such effector cells are capable of mediating regression of established small and large tumors located in visceral organs, although their effects seem to be more limited in subcutaneously located tumors [11]. The combined anti-tumoral effect of LAK- cell transfer and high dose injections of IL-2 is not attenuated by whole-body x-ray irradiation, supporting the view that immunesurveillance is not critical for the effect, as confirmed in animal experiments [12]. It has also been reported that human tumors are associated with circulating serum factor(s) that can inhibit the induction of the LAK cell activation, and subsequent surgical removal of the tumors restored the induction completely [13]. This may be a significant observation, which is distinct from other inhibitors in autologous serum from cancer patients. Such factors generally inhibited the effector reaction (cytolysis) *in vitro*.

Several hundred patients have so far been treated with adoptive immunotherapy. It is, however, disputed whether these efforts have presented any therapeutical benefit that is not achieved by conventional chemotherapy or conventional combined treatment modalities at a much lower cost [14]. A major limitation, so far, has been the toxicity of high-dose IL-2 infusions [15]. Locoregional administration routes such as locoinfusion directly into the brain in patients with gliomas, and intraperitoneally to patients with carcinosis, may limit the toxic reactions [16].

Interleukines

There are at present 6 well-defined interleukines with known amino-acid sequences. All these molecules have been cloned and are available as recombinant forms with metabolic and cellular effects that probably are very similar to those of the naturally occurring substances. The molecular characterization of these substances, including sequence determination, have revealed that many previously described substances or recently reported bioactivities (with different names) in test systems can actually be ascribed to identical or nearly identical molecules. For example, lymphocyte activating factor (LAF) and leukocyte endogenous mediator (LEM) turned out to be identical to interleukin 1 (IL-1). Hepatocyte stimulating factor (HPS) and interferon beta-2 were found to be identical and were named interleukin 6 (IL-6). The interleukines are produced in many different cell types such as macrophages, monocytes, lymphocytes, reticulo-endothelial cells, vascular endothelial cells, fibroblasts and also in various progenitor cells in blood forming cell lines.

There are also a number of classical growth factors, such as transforming growth factor alpha and beta (TGF alpha, beta), granulocyte and macrophage colony stimulating factors (CSFs), platelet derived growth factor (PDGF), epidermal growth factor (EGF), which appear to interact with signal peptides in parts of the immune system. Most recently it has also become evident that many of these signal peptides and growth factors also interact directly or indirectly with the classical hormone system as well as with the nervous system [17-20]. Such effector and feed-back pathways illustrate a very complex integration of many cellular, regulating and communicating systems both within and outside the immune system.

Tumor necrosis factor (TNF-alpha) is a macrophage-derived molecule also named cachectin, due to its well-recognized "catabolic" effects in both humans and animals [21,22]. TNF-beta is a lymphotoxin derived from lymphocytes with less well recognized effects than TNF-alpha, although most of its examined effects are similar or identical to that of TNF. Tumor necrosis factor and lymphotoxin bear approximately 30% sequence homology and are closely linked to TNF on chromosome 6. The sequence homology is around 80% conserved between man, mouse and rabbit. TNF-alpha, which has a molecular weight of 17,000 dalton, containing to residues linked by a disulfide bond, was first identified in view of its anticancer activity in some animal models. [23-25]. TNF is now suggested to be one of a family of proteins that orchestrate the host's response to injury and infection. TNF is different from IL-1 in structure but shares many effects in the host with IL-1. TNF stimulates granulocytes to be adhesive to endothelial cells and to produce toxic oxygen products that destroy bacteria. TNF along with IL-1 also activates T lymphocytes to IL-2 receptor expression and to subsequent IL-2 production. Class-I MHC antigen expression is increased in fibroblast and endothelial cells following addition of TNF. Both TNF and IL-1 act on the thermoregulatory center in the brain to produce fever [26,27]. Preliminary results suggest that this effect is in part mediated by both the classical hormone system and the neuroendocrine response, which activates brown adipose tissue thermogenesis. In this respect IL-1beta and TNF seem to be different in the sense that the IL-1-beta effect is dependent on the production of hypothalamic corticotrophic hormone (CRF) [28]. Another effect, the increased synthesis of acute phase proteins, is in part an indirect result of TNF; the hepatic synthesis of many acute phase proteins is regulated by the recently described interleukin-6 [29,30]

One of the most prominent effects of TNF is its regulation of the enzyme lipoprotein lipase activity in different tissues such as fat cells and liver cells. "Cachectin" was actually discovered by this regulation, a function that it shares with IL-1 and interferon gamma. The role of these cytokines and other factors in causing cachexia in patients with chronic infection and cancer has been suggested elsewhere by ourselves [31] and others [18], but the mechanisms are far from clear. In addition, the effect of TNF to induce hemorrhage and necrosis in tumor tissue is also not well understood. Beyond its effect to stimulate immune cells against tumor cells, there seems to be a more immediate effect on tumors. In animal experiments TNF was shown to destroy the blood vessel supply of the tumor [32,33]. In contrast to malignant tissue, TNF seems to stimulate neovascularisation to untransformed cells, a characteristic it shares with at least 4 other cytokines. It has also been reported that TNF may exert cell-killing under conditions when certain normal cell functions are not acting normally, such as an impaired RNA or protein synthesis. This effect may also occur in cells that do not respond to TNF under normal conditions. What actually causes such cytocidal effects is unclear, but it may be that TNF activates intracellular enzymes liberating highly reactive molecules that injure and finally kill the cells.

Circulating levels of TNF have not consistently been found in cancer patients but may be more generally found in severely infected patients [34,35]. There is no natural inhibitor to TNF in the circulation as there is for IL-1. Only few cancer patients have shown any objective response to intravenous injections or infusions of TNF only as single-drug therapy. With direct injections of TNF into human tumors some response was observed.

The infusion of TNF to dogs at doses that could be produced during bacteremia stimulate progressive hemodynamic collapse, shock and death [36]. The metabolic response is characterized by elevation of catecholamines, cortisol and glucagon. Acute inflammation of the lungs, acute renal tubular necrosis and hemorrhagic adrenal glands are seen at autopsy. Cellular metabolism is characterized by energy mobilization, lactate production, elevated glucose transport and glycogen depletion concomitant with changes in the cellular membrane potentials. All these effects cannot, however, be ascribed directly to TNF. Although bowel necrosis induced by TNF is indistinguishable from that produced by endotoxin and can be blocked by anti-TNF, it is now known that platelet activating factor (PAF) is also an causative agent with additive effects to endotoxin and TNF [37].

Interleukin-1 is synthesized in two molecular forms (alpha and beta) as a pre-protein with an approximate molecular weight of 32,000 dalton. It is processed by tryptic cleavage to a 17,000 dalton protein when leaving the cell, as are most "export proteins". The homology sequence is only 30% between the two molecular forms, but the interspecies homology seems to be better conserved and is around 70% in eucaryotic cells [38]. This means that the human recombinant form can be used in animal experiments and can give meaningful qualitative and semiquantitative information. IL-1 can be detected in plasma if the naturally occurring inhibitor is first eliminated. IL-1 beta is the predominantly circulating form, while it has been suggested that IL-1 alpha may be the predominantly cellular form, perhaps exerting its major effects when bound to the cellular membrane of the producing cells. IL-1 is rarely found at increased levels in patients with acute phase responses, although it has been demonstrated in patients with acute bacterial infections. Therefore, the main effect of IL-1 is its being a paracrinic hormone in different cell tissue compartments. IL-1 is produced by a variety of cells within and outside the immune system. It is one of the major inducers of fever, acute phase protein synthesis, trace metal redistribution from plasma, anemia secondary to inflammation and infection. Due to all these effects it has been called the hormone of inflammation. In addition to these effects, IL-1 has distinct effects on T-cells, B-cells including immunoglobulin synthesis and on natural killer cells. In this regard, IL-1 has both stimulatory and sensitizing effects that are very complex and multifunctional.

Interleukin-2 is a substance that has been widely used in therapeutical efforts to stimulate and sensitize lymphocytes and killer cells and is mainly produced by helper T-cells. IL-2 is a T-cell growth factor, which binds to the IL-2 receptor on T-cells eliciting the subsequent clonal expansion of particularly killer T-cells, but may also stimulate suppressor T-cells. IL-2 is a 15,500-dalton protein with varying glyco- and sialoglycosylation. Its tertiary structure seems to be important for its effect on the receptor, which is both a high affinity and a low affinity receptor population [39]. Recombinant IL-2 to mice increases secondary alloimmune responses, enhances NK activity and may generate LAK cell activity, at least with high doses. *In vivo* administration of IL-2 has, however, shown a rapid disappearance from the circulation, emphasizing the limited effects that can be achieved, even with high-dose injections [15]. This is particularly evident in the light of its severe side effects, such as fluid retention, vomiting, nausea, headache, fever, malaise, diarrhea, occasional rash with pruritus and even respiratory insufficiency. Most of these side effects, except for the fluid retention, can be blocked or attenuated by indomethacin. The presence of IL-2 in biological fluids can be demonstrated by either bioassays or radioimmunoassays [40].

Interleukin 3 is the same as multi-CSF (see below).

Interleukin 4 is a potent mast cell growth factor originally identified by its ability to enhance proliferation of B lymphocytes [41,42].

Interleukin 5 is the eosinophil differentiation factor [43]. The molecule stimulates the formation of eosinophils which are particularly adapted for killing parasites. This is an antibody-dependent process. The gene is quite small and code for the protein which is 134 amino acids, corresponding to a molecular weight of around 15,000 dalton. The human and murine sequences are approx. 70% identical. IL-5 is probably produced by activated T-lymphocytes.

Interleukin 6 is mainly produced by monocytes. Much weaker sources of IL-6 production are fibroblasts, smooth muscle and endothelial cells. The molecule was originally described as a hybridoma B-cell growth factor (HGF), with a molecular weight of 21-25,000 dalton. The sequence of HGF was subsequently found to be identical with that described for interferon-beta 2 [44], as well as to the sequence of BSF-2, a B cell differentiation factor reported by Hirano et al. [45]; it is also identical to the hepatocyte stimulation factor (HSF). For this molecule the name interleukin-6 was proposed. The gene has been cloned and recent experiments show that rIL-6 has very similar effects to IL-1 and TNF-alpha *in vivo*, and is now suggested to be the major and most important molecule to stimulate the synthesis of hepatic acute phase proteins [29]. It may even be expected that many of the systemic effects of either IL-1 or TNF may actually be ascribed to IL-6 in the near future. Our own experiments have demonstrated large quantities of IL-6 in the circulation of tumor-bearing animals with acute phase response, but without detectable IL-1 or TNF levels [46].

IL-6 acts predominantly on resting T-cells, but this effect is fundamentally different from that of IL-2, which acts by stimulation of the IL-2 receptor on the T-cells.

Interferons

The interferons are a family of proteins that are primarily characterized by their ability to prevent and attenuate virus replication. The interferons do not cross-react among species. Interferon-alpha, which is produced by leucocytes or NK-like lymphocytes, has been used for many years in clinical trials of cancer treatment [47]. Although the therapeutical effects have been limited in most applications, some tumor forms seem to respond. The best example of this is probably hairy-cell leukemia [48].

Beta-interferon is produced by fibroblasts. Gamma-interferon is produced by antigen-stimulated lymphocytes and has been found to greatly enhance the effect of cytokines on immune cells, inhibiting the proliferation of some tumor cells and inducing the expression of HLA class-II antigens in tumors, which may be weak in many patients and animals. The interferons, particularly the alpha and beta forms, have also been demonstrated to attenuate or inhibit cell proliferation induced by growth factors such as platelet-derived growth factor [49]. Due to the profound sensitizing effect on various progenitor and mature immune cells, gamma-interferon will most probably gain interest and importance as an adjunct substance in many research and clinical protocols for the treatment of cancer in the near future.

Growth Factors

A new family of polypeptide factors that regulate cell growth and differentiation has emerged [50]. Transforming growth factor beta (TGF-beta), a 25,000-dalton disulfide-linked homodimer, originally found in transformed fibroblasts, is the prototype of these proteins, and is now emerging as one of the most interesting and significant growth factor molecules. This family of proteins interacts with cell proliferation and differentiation in various cell types. They can also modulate differentiated functions in lymphocytes, granulosa and adrenocortical cells and act in the regulation of matrix turnover.
Transforming growth factor alpha (TGF-alpha) is secreted by a variety of human and rodent tumors and can induce the "reversible transformation" of non-transformed or normal cell lines by stimulating growth and anchorage independence. TGF-alpha competes with the epidermal growth factor (EGF) receptor [51]. Large amounts of various forms of peptides belonging to the TGF-alpha family have been demonstrated in tumor tissue samples and urine from cancer patients with many common solid tumor types [52-54].
The regulated production of blood cells is one of the most complex examples of multilineage cell differentiation under the control of the 4 myeloid growth factors called colony stimulating factors (CSFs): granulocyte colony stimulating factor (G-CSF), granulocyte-macrophage colony stimulating factor (GM-CSF), multi-CSF also called interleukin-3 (IL-3), and macrophage colony stimulating factor (M-CSF) [55].

G-CSF is a lineage-specific factor that directly supports proliferation of cell colonies consisting of neutrophils. It also enhances the ability of neutrophils to produce superoxide anions and facilitate chemotaxis and phagocytosis. G-CSF is a growth and differentiation factor for late progenitor cells committed to the neutrophil lineage.
GM-CSF supports the proliferation of macrophage and eosinophil cell colonies as well as colonies containing both macrophages and neutrophils. It interacts with earlier progenitors than G-CSF does. GM-CSF is also a survival and activating factor for the end cell derived from GM-CSF progenitors. Thus, it enhances the activities of neutrophils, macrophages and eosinophils.
Multi-CSF (IL-3) supports the proliferation of myeloid progenitors including those of erythrocytes, eosinophils, basophils, macrophages and megakaryocytes and probably also neutrophils.
M-CSF is capable of activating mature macrophages and it probably functions as a survival and activating factor for monocytes and macrophages in addition to enhancing macrophage cytotoxicity. The identification of the M-CSF receptor as the gene product of the *fms* protooncogene is of great interest.

These myeloid growth factors have already been or will soon be subjected to clinical trials. They were found to have an unexpectedly low toxicity in phase I and II clinical trials, and to stimulate bone marrow production *in vivo* in humans according to their experimentally defined activities in cell cultures and monkeys. Leukopenic patients with AIDS or following chemotherapy have responded extremely well. This fact may create a new therapeutical approach in bone marrow transplantation and perhaps in blood production before surgery. The recent discovery that cytokines, particularly IL-1 and TNF, stimulate the production of these myeloid growth factors in both T-lymphocytes and fibroblasts, demonstrates new links between progenitors and effector cells on activation to combat threats. Colony stimulating factors may thus provide additional facilities to expand the tumor treatment potential in the near future, in combination with cytokine activation.

Multifunctional Effects of Cytokines *In Vivo*

Monokines and lymphokines have, thus, gained increasing interest over the past years as biological response modifiers in the treatment of various malignant tumors, but also in the research on cachexia, infection, trauma and shock. This is true in particular for the lymphokine interleukin-2 and the cytokines IL-1 and TNF. It is already obvious that no single molecule can be responsible for the whole spectrum of events that are necessary to extinguish malignant cells from the host for cure or to explain the induction and promotion of cachexia and shock.

Monokines and Anorexia

It has been observed by others and by ourselves that the presence of antigens may stimulate macrophages, perhaps both circulatory and resident, to excrete substances that will depress food intake [56-58]. It is obvious that stimulated macrophages will upregulate the production of numerous different proteins of which few or several may have this anorectic effect. Figure 1 demonstrates that some of these molecules may well be interleukin-1 and tumor necrosis factor (TNF-alpha), as confirmed by the injection of these recombinant gene products of both murine and human origin. However, it is unclear whether these substances exert their effect directly or indirectly on the appetite-regulating regions in the central nervous system. The answer to this question must await additional experiments, although the presence and the expression of interleukin-1 receptors have been demonstrated in brain tissue [59,60]. Recent suggestions and brief reports have emphasized that interleukin-6 is also involved in one way or another [61]. One model may be that either IL-1, TNF or the two of them stimulate immune cells to secrete IL-6, which is the circulating communicating message to the brain in an immune-stressed animal. In the brain either IL-6 or some other monokines, perhaps the local production of IL-1 or TNF, may stimulate its own receptor(s). Unfortunately, we have not been able so far to demonstrate a significant upregulation of mRNA synthesis for either TNF or IL-1 in brain tissue from stressed and tumor-bearing animals suffering from severe anorexia. Recent results, however, demonstrate that intraventricular injections of IL-6 will produce similar changes in appetite, energy balance, thermogenesis and fever as IL-1 and TNF [62].

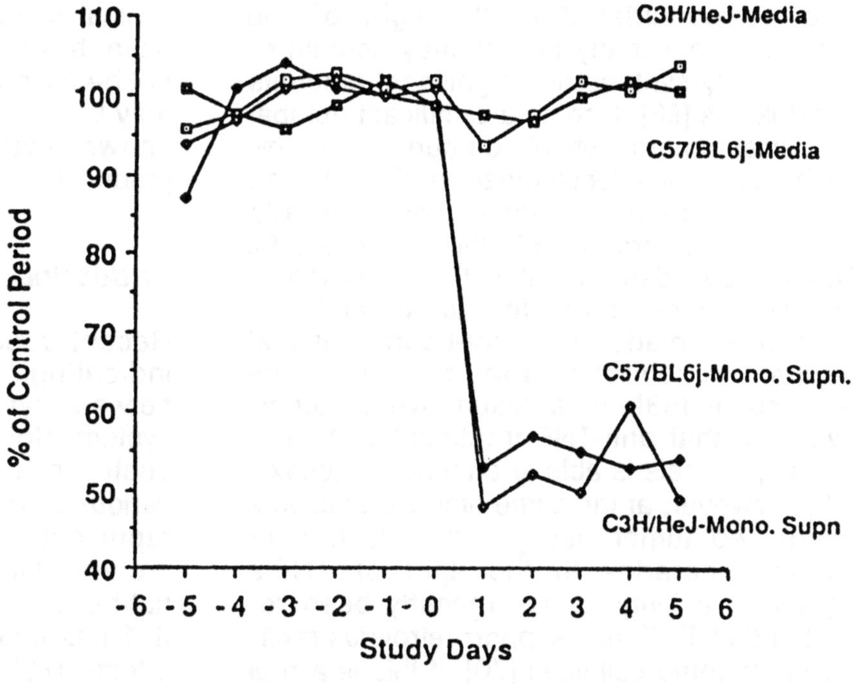

Fig. 1. Food intake in mice given soluble products of activated blood monocytes. C3H/Hej mice are resistant to the metabolic effects of endotoxin. C57Bl mice are sensitive to the metabolic effects of endotoxin and the products that are released after stimulating blood monocytes with endotoxin (Staphylococcus albus). "Media" refers to monocytic products that are derived from cell culture medium following incubation of monocytes, and "supernatant" refers to products derived from the supernatant following lysis of the incubated monocytes

Evidence has recently been reported that TNF inhibits tumor growth *in vivo* by interfering with the vascular supply to the tumor [63]. However, in the evaluation of various results from *in vivo* studies on the effect of monokines on tumor growth, it is important to remember that experimental tumors are extremely sensitive to metabolic substrate supplies. The simplest way to decrease or inhibit tumor cell proliferation may just be to decrease the food intake of the animal. This may lead to altered cell cycle kinetics within hours, and refeeding may then reinduce proliferation. Considering the strong anorectic effect of many cytokines, it is thus necessary to account for such factors by pair-feeding experimental animals before any conclusion can be drawn with respect to the specific tumor inhibition by cytokines in specific experiments. This was not done in the majority of the published reports on monokines, experimental immunomodulation and tumor growth. Whether similar effects have any bearing on the clinical situation remains to be seen, but undernutrition and refeeding can influence the cell cycle kinetics also in human tumors [64,65]. In addition, ongoing trials with cytokine injection should also be considered in the light of the possibility that many tumors may contain or are actually synthesizing significant amounts of cytokines [66]. If so, in a significant number of clinical tumors it should be questioned how such exogenous recombinant molecules can have therapeutical effects when already endogenously produced in the tumor [67,68]. Others have demonstrated that insertion of the TNF-alpha gene into tumor cells by transfection made the tumor-bearing animal become cachectic due to TNF-gene expression [68]. In addition, we obtained evidence that anti-TNF treatment to tumor-bearing animals is able to attenuate cachexia [69]. However, at the same time we noticed a decreased tumor net growth, which may seem a paradox in the light of TNF's antitumor activity. It has recently been reported that TNF may support retrovirus replication in some cell lines [70]. If this is a real observation, it may represent a problem in future clinical studies.

Metabolic Effects of Monokines

Cytokines such as IL-1 and TNF have profound metabolic effects, although again it is not clear whether such effects are secondary to their immune and acute phase reactions. The most well-recognized effect is that of TNF-alpha to regulate the enzyme lipoprotein lipase in fat cells [71]. This effect has been suggested to explain or at least contribute to the elevation of free fatty acids in stress conditions, i.e., to mobilize the fat substrate for oxidation. TNF also seems to have adrenergic influences in brown fat in animals, and both IL-1 and TNF stimulate energy expenditure in both man and animals beside mechanisms that are not only dependent on their fever-inducing effects in the hypothalamus. It is, however, not quite clear to what extent these effects are primary or secondary to activation of other cytokines. Likewise it was originally reported that IL-1 induced prostaglandines in skeletal muscles, which led to the activation of protein breakdown of muscle proteins [72]. It was, therefore, suggested that IL-1 was the major inducing substance behind muscle wasting in several clinical conditions. More recent experiments have, however, revealed that this effect cannot be ascribed to either IL-1 or TNF [73], but may be the effect of some other perhaps unknown cytokine or macrophage-derived product [74].

Endocrine Effects

Recent research has provided evidence indicating a very complex interaction between cytokines and the classical hormone system. So far it is not clear to what extent such an endocrine interplay represents various physiological pathways or may rather represent endocrinological side effects that are well-documented experimentally but may not be that important in the *in vivo* situation. IL-1 has many levels of endocrine regulatory effects [75]. It may promote the release of hypothalamic factors that can stimulate the release of pituitary hormones, directly activate the pituitary gland and thereby indirectly activate the adrenals, particularly the secretion of glucocorticoids. It has also been demonstrated that IL-1 has a direct receptor-mediated function on the adrenals to produce corticosteroids [76]. Our own investigations and those of others have demonstrated that the adrenals have a permissive action for the effect of IL-1 to support part of the response, namely the hepatic synthesis of at least some of the acute-phase proteins (unpublished results). The toxic dose level is also severely lowered in adrenalectomized animals, which may have some influence on the clinical situation. This effect is not similar for TNF. Such discrepancies between two related and simultaneously produced molecules upon macrophage stimulation demonstrate a very complex positive and negative feed-back regulation of cytokine production and their target effects. The permissive effect of glucocorticoids for part of the IL-1 effect is particularly interesting in the light of the well-known fact that glucocorticoids on the other hand can attenuate or completely block parts of the cytokine cascade effect [77]. Results have also been reported that support the suggestion that monokines, particularly IL-1, can destroy the beta-cells in the pancreas under some conditions, which may be of significance for the onset of diabetes, perhaps in combination with viral infections [78].

Considering all the effects that are already known to be exerted by cytokines, at the interorgan and at the cellular level, it is very unlikely that we will ever learn to predict or understand in detail what will happen in clinical trials where recombinant cytokines and antigenically stimulated cells are artificially produced and then adoptively introduced into the host. The therapeutical benefits and the degree of side effects will continue to be learned mainly on empirical grounds, but our basic knowledge on the host effects of monokines will certainly continue to grow rapidly.

REFERENCES

1 Hericourt J and Richet CCR: hebd. Seanc. Acad. Sci 1895 (121): 567.
2 Ngu VA: In: Burchenal JH and Burkitt D (eds) Treatment of Burkitt's Lymphoma. Springer, New York 1967 p 204
3 Nadler SH, Moore GE: Immunotherapy of malignant disease. Arch Surg 1969 (99):376-381
4 Andrews GA, Congdon CC, Edwards CL, Gengozian N, Nelson B, Vodopick H: Preliminary trials of clinical immunotherapy. Cancer Res 1967 (27):2535-2541
5 Trouillas P, Lapras C: Cellular immunotherapy of cerebral glioblastoma. A propos of 2 results. J Med Lyon 1969 (50):1269-1291
6 Yron I, Wood TA, Spiess P, Rosenberg SA: In vitro growth of murine T cells: V The isolation and growth of lymphoid cell infiltrating syngeneic solid tumors. J Immunol 1980 (125):238-245
7 Lotze MT, Grimme E, Mazumder A, Strausser JL, Rosenberg SA: In vitro growth of cytotoxic human lymphocytes, IV. Lysis of fresh and cultured autologous tumor by lymphocytes cultured in T cell growth factor (TCGF). Cancer Res 1981 (41):4420-4425
8 Grimm EA, Mazumder A, Zang HZ, Rosenberg SA: The lymphokine activated killer cell phenomenon: Lysis of NK resistant fresh solid tumor cells by IL-2 activated autoloogous human peripheral blood lymphocytes. J Exp Med 1982 (155):1823-1851
9 Grimm EA, Ramsey KM, Mazumder A, Wilson DJ, Djeu JY, Rosenberg SA: Lymphokine activated killer cell phenomenon: II The precursor phenotype is serologically distinct from peripherals T lymphocytes, memory CTL, and NK cells. J Exp Med 1983 (157):884-897
10 Rosenstein M, Yron I , Kaufman Y, Rosenberg SA: Lympokine-activated killer cells: Lysis of fresh syngeneic NK-resistant murine tumor cells by lymphocytes cultured in interleukin-2. Cancer Res 1984 (44):1946-1953
11 Mule JJ, Shu S, Schwarz SL, Rosenberg SA: Successful adoptive immunotherapy of established pulmonary metastases with lymphokine-activated killer cells and recombinant interleukin-2. Science 1984 (225):1487
12 Rosenberg SA, Mulé JJ: mmunotheraphy of cancer with lymphokine-activated killer cells and recombinant interleukin-2. Surgery 1985 (98):437-444
13 Balch CM, Itoh K, Tilden AB: Cellular immune defects in patients with melanoma involving interleukin-2-activated lymphocyte cytotoxicity and a serum suppressor factor. Surgery 1985 (98):151-157
14 Grimm EA: Immunotherapy of advanced cancer. N Engl Med 1987 (316):275-276
15 Lotze MT, Matory YL, Ettinghausen SE, Rayner AA, Sharow S, Seipp C, Custer M, Rosenberg SA: In vivo administration of purified human interleukin-2 II. Half life, Immunologic effects, and expansion of peripheral lymphoid cells in vivo with recombinant IL-2. J Immunol 1985 (135):2865-2875
16 Jacobs SK, Wilson DJ, Kornblith PL, Grimm E: Interleukin-2 or autologous lymphokine-activated cell treatment of malignant glioma:Phase I trial. Cancer Res 1986 (46):2101-2104
17 Besedovsky H, Del Rey A, Sorkin E, Dinarello CA: Immunoregulatory feedback between interleukin 1 and glucocorticoid hormones. Science (USA) 1986 (233):652-654
18 Dinarello CA: An update on human interleukin-1: from molecular biology to clinical relevance. J Clin Immunol 1985 (5):287-297
19 Roh MS, Drazenovich KA, Barbose JJ, Dinarello CA, Cobb CF: Direct stimulation of the adrenal cortex by interleukin-1. Surgery 1987 (102):140-146
20 Coombes RC, Rothwell NJ, Shah P, Stock MJ: Changes in thermogenesis and brown fat activity in response to tumour necrosis factor in the rat. Bioscience Reports 1987 (7):791-799
21 Beutler B, Cerami A: Cachectin and tumour necrosis factor as two sides of the same biological coin. Nature 1986 (320):584-588
22 Tracey KJ, Lowry SF, Fahey III TJ, Albert JD, Fong Y, Hesse D, Beutler B, Manogue KR, Calvano S, Wei H, Cerami A, Shires GT: Cachectin-tumor necrosis factor induces lethal shock and stress hormone responses in the dog. Surg Gynecol Obstet 1987 (164):415-422
23 Carswell EA, Old LJ, Kassel RL, Green S, Fiore N, Williamson B: An endotoxin induced serum factor that causes necrosis of tumors. Proc Natl Acad Sci (USA) 1975 (72):3666-3670
24 Haranaki K, Carswell EA, Williamson BD, Prendegast JS, Satomi N, Old LJ: Purification, characterization and antitumour activity of nonrecombinant mouse tumour necrosis factor. Proc Natl Acad Sci (USA) 1986 (83):3949-3953
25 Old LJ: Tumor necrosis factor. Scientific American 1988 (25):41-49
26 Nishimura T, Ohta S, Sato N, Togashi Y, Goto M, Hashimoto Y: Combination tumor-immunotherapy with recombinant tumor necrosis factor and recombinant interleukin 2 in mice. Int J Cancer 1987 (40):255-261
27 Bodel P: Tumours and fever. Ann NY Acad Sci 1974 (230):6-13
28 Coombes RC, Rothwell NJ, Shah P, Stock MJ: Changes in thermogenesis and brown fat activity in response to tumour necrosis factor in the rat. Bioscience Reports 1987 (7):791-799
29 Baumann H, Richards C, Gauldie J: Interaction among hepatocyte-stimulating factors, interleukin-1, and glucocorticoids for regulation of acute phase plasma proteins in human hepatoma (HepG2) cells. J Immunol 1987 (139):4122-4128
30 Walther Z, May LT, Sehgal PB: Transcriptional regulation of the interferon-B2-B cell differentiation factor BSF-2-Hepatocyte-stimulating factor gene in human fibroblasts by other cytokines. J Immunol 1988 (140):974-977
31 Moldawer LL, Georgieff M, Lundholm K: Interleukin 1, tumour necrosis factor-alpha (cachectin) and the pathogenesis of cancer cachexia. Clin Physiol 1987 (7):263-274
32 Havell E, Fiers W, North R J: The antitumor function of tumor necrosis factor (TNF). I. Therapeutic action

of TNF against an established murine sarcoma is indirect, immunologically dependent, and limited by severe toxicity. J Exp Med 1988 (167):1067-1085
33 North RJ, Havell EA: The antitumor function of tumor necrosis factor (TNF). II. Analysis of the role of endogenous TNF in endotoxin-induced hemorrhagic necrosis and regression of an established sarcoma. J Exp Med 1988 (167):1086-1099
34 Waage A, Espevik T, Lamvik J: Detection of tumour necrosis factor-like cytotoxicity in serum from patients with septicaemia but not from untreated cancer patients. Scand J Immunol 1986 (24):739-743
35 Balkwill F, Osborne R, Burke F, Naylor S, Talbot D, Durbin H, Tavernier J, Fiers W: Evidence for tumour necrosis factor-cachectin production in cancer. Lancet 1987 (2):1229-1232
36 Tracey KJ, Lowry SF, Fahey III TJ, Albert JD, Fong Y, Hesse D, Beutler B, Manogue KR, Calvano S, Wei H, Cerami A, Shires GT: Cachectin-tumor necrosis factor induces lethal shock and stress hormone responses in the dog. Surg Gynecol Obstet 1987 (164):415-422
37 Sun XM, Hsueh W: Bowel necrosis induced by tumor necrosis factor in rats is mediated by platelet-activating factor. J Clin Invest 1988 (81):1328-1331
38 Dinarello CA: Interleukin 1. Rev Infect Dis 1984 (6):51-94
39 Hakim AA: Peripheral blood lymphocytes from patients with cancer lack interleukin-2 receptors. Cancer 1988 (61):689-701
40 Ferrua B, Aussel C, Fehlman M: Human interleukin 2. Detection at the picomolar level by sandwich enzyme immunoassay. Journal of Immunological Methods 1987 (97):215-220
41 Lee F, Yokota T, Otsuka T, Meyerson P, Villaret D, Coffman R, Mosmann T, Rennick D, Roehm N, Smith C et al: Isolation and characterization of a mouse interleukin cDNA clone that expresses B-cell stimulatory factor 1 activities and T-cell- and mast cell-stimulating activities. Proc Natl Acad Sci USA 1986 (83):2061-2065
42 Hamaguchi Y, Kanakura Y, Fujita J, Takeda S, Nakano T, Tarui S, Honjo T, Kitamura Y: Interleukin 4 as an essential factor for in vitro clonal growth of murine connective tissue-type mast cells. J Exp Med 1987 (165):268-273
43 Campbell HD, Tucker WQJ, Hort Y, Martinson ME, Mayo G, Clutterbuck EJ, Sanderson CJ, Young IG: Molecular cloning, nucleotide sequence, and expression of the gene encoding human eosinophil differentiation factor (interleukin 5). Proc Natl Acad Sci USA 1987 (84):6629-6633
44 Koj A, Gordon AH, Gauldie J: An alternative regulatory pathway of the acute phase response: the role of fibroblast-derived interferon-beta 2. Experientia 1988 (44):9-10
45 Hirano T, Yasukawa K, Harada H, Tage T, Yasuo W, Matsuda T, Kishiwamure S, Nakajima K, Koyama K, Wamatsu A, Tsunasawa S, Sakiyama F, Matsui H, Takahara Y, Taniguchi T, Kishimoto T: Complementary DNA for a novel human interleukin (BSF-2) that induces B lymphocytes to produce immunoblobulin. Nature 1986 (324):73
46 Gelin J, Moldawer L, Lönnroth C, DeMan P, Svanborg-Eden C, Lowry S, Lundholm K: Appearence of hybridoma growth factor/interleukin 6 in the serum of cachectic mice bearing a methylcholantrene induced sarcoma. Submitted for publication
47 Goldstein D, Laszlo J: Interferon therapy in cancer: From Imaginon to Interferon. Cancer Res 1986 (46):4315-4329
48 Aderka D, Levo Y, Ramot B, Michalevicz R, Meytes D, Shaklai M, Hahn T, Holtmann H, Revel M, Wallach D: Reduced production of tumor necrosis factor by mononuclear cells in hairy cell leukemia patients and improvement following interferon therapy. Cancer 1987 (60):2208-2212
49 Einat M, Resnitzky D, Kimchi A: Inhibitory effects of interferon on genes regulated by platlet-derived growth factor. Proc Natl Acad Sci USA 1985 (82):7608-7612
50 Massagué J: The TGF-ß family of growth factors and differentiation factors: Minireview. Cell 1987 (49):437-438
51 Sclessinge J, Schreiber A, Levi A, Lax I, Liberman T, Yarden Y: Regulation of cell proliferation by epidermal growth factor. Critical Review in Biochemistry 1983 (14):93-111
52 Nickell KA, Halper J, Moses H: Transforming growth factors in solid human malignant neoplasms. Cancer Res 1983 (43):1966-1971
53 Kimball ES, Bohn WH, Cockley KD, Warren TC, Sherwin SA: Distinct high-performance liquid chromatography pattern of transforming growth factor activity in urine of cancer patients as compared with that of normal individuals. Cancer Res 1984 (44):3613-3619
54 Sherwin SA, Twardzik DR, Bohn WH, Cockley KC, Todaro GJ: High-molecular-weight transforming growth factor activity in the urine of patients with disseminated cancer. Cancer Res 1983 (43):403-407
55 Clark SC, Kamen R: The human hematopoietic colony-stimulating factors. Science 1987 (236):1229-1237
56 Morrison SD: Control of food intake in cancer cachexia. A challenge and a tool. Pysiol Behav 1976 (17):705 - 714
57 Moldawer LL, Andersson C, Gelin J, Lundholm KG: Regulation of food intake and hepatic protein synthesis by recombinant-derived cytokines. Am J Physiol 1988 (254):450-456
58 McCarthey DO, Kluger MJ, Vander AJ: Suppression of food intake during infection: is interleukin 1 involved?.Amer J Clin Nutr 1985 (42):1179-1182
59 Dinarello CA, Bernheim HA: Ability of human leukocytic pyrogen to stimulate brain prostaglandin synthesis in vitro. J Neurochem 1981 (37):702-708
60 Giulian D, Lachman LB: Interleukin 1 stimulation of astroglial cell proliferation after brain injury. Science (USA) 1985 (228):497-499
61 Houssiau FA, Bukasa K, Sindic CJM, Van Damme J, Van Snick J: Elevated levels of 26K human hybridoma growth factor (interleukin 6) in cerebrospinal fluid of patients with acute infection of the central nervous system. Clin Exp Immunol 1988 (71):320-323

62 Busbridge J, Dascombe MJ, Hoopkins S, Rothwell NJ: Acute central effects of interleukin-6 on body temperature, thermogenesis and food intake in the rat. In press 1988
63 Shimomura K, Manda T, Mukumoto S, Kobayashi K, Nakano K, Mori J: recombinant human tumor necrosis factor-a: Thrombus formation is a cause of anti-tumor activity. Int J Cancer 1988 (41):243-247
64 Baron PL, Lawrence W Jr, Chan WMY, White FKH, Banks WL: Effects of parenteral nutrition on cell cycle kinetics of head and neck cancer. Arch Surg 1986 (121):1282-1286
65 Edström S, Westin T, Delle U, Lundholm K: Cell cycle distribution and ornithine decarboxylase activity in head and neck cancer in response to enteral nutrition. Eur J Cancer Clin Oncol1988 (in press)
66 Lönnroth C, Moldawer L, Gelin J, Kindblom LG, Mizel B, Lundholm G: Spontaneous interleukin-1-alpha and cachectin production by tumor cell of cachectic tumor-bearing mice. J. Exper Med. In press 1988
67 Duncombe AS, Gottlieb DJ, Bianchi A, Brenner MK: Bioactivity and immunoreactivity of tumor necrosis factor in cancer patients:.letter to the Editor. Lancet 1988 (Januari 30):248
68 Oliff A, Defeo-Jones D, Boyer M, Martinez D, Kiefer D, Vuocolo G, Wolfe A, Socher SH: Tumors secreting human TNF-cachectin induce cachexia in mice. Cell 1987 (50):555-563
69 Sherry BA, Gelin J, Fong Y, Marano M, Wei H, Cerami A, Lowry S, Lundholm K, Moldawer L: Anticachectin/tumor necrosis factor-alpha antibodies attenuate the development of cachexia in two murine transplantable tumor models. Submitted for publication 1988
70 Yagi MJ, Holland JF, Bekesi JG: Tumor necrosis factor enhances murine SL3-3 retrovirus replication. J Clin Lab Immunol 1987 (24):129-134
71 Kawakami M, Cerami A: Studies of endotoxin induced decrease in lipoprotein lipase activity. J Exp Med 1981 (154):631-637
72 Baracos V, Rodemann HP, Dinarello CA, Goldberg AL: Stimulation of muscle protein degradation and prostaglandin E2 release by leukocytic pyrogen (Interleukin 1). New Engl J Med 1983 (308):553-558
73 Moldawer LL, Svaninger G, Gelin J, Lundholm K: Interleukin-1 (alpha or beta) and tumor necrosis factor alpha do not regulate protein balance in skeletal muscle. Am J Physiol 1987 (253):C766-C773
74 Goldberg AL, Kettelhut IC, Furuno K, Fagan JM, Baracos V: Activation of protein breakdown and prostaglandin E2 production in rat skeletal muscle in fever is signaled by a macrophage product distinct from interleukin 1 or other known monokines. J Clin Invest 1988 (81):1378-1383
75 Hill MR, Stith RD, McCallum RE: Interleukin 1: a regulatory role in glucocorticoid regulated hepatic metabolism. J Immunol 1986 (137):858-862
76 Roh MS, Drazenovich KA, Barbose JJ, Dinarello CA, Cobb CF: Direct stimulation of the adrenal cortex by interleukin-1. Surgery 1987 (102):140-146
77 Knudsen PJ, Dinarello CA, Strom TB: Glucocorticoids inhibit transcriptional and posttranscriptional expression of interleukin 1 in U937 cells. J Immunol 1987 (139):4129 - 4134
78 Mandrup-Poulsen T, Bendtzen K, Dinarello CA, Nerup J: Human tumor necrosis factor potentiates human interleukin 1-mediated rat pancreatic beta-cell cytotoxicity. J Immunol 1987 (139):4077-4082

The Rationale of Intraarterial Chemotherapy of Liver Cancer

P. Schlag and P. Hohenberger

Section of Surgical Oncology, Department of Surgery, University of Heidelberg, 6900 Heidelberg, Germany

Introduction

The rationale of regional chemotherapy in malignant liver tumours is based on an increased drug uptake in the tumour tissue, while at the same time the side effects of the therapy are reduced. Although nearly 40 years ago the theoretical treatment concept was already discussed in detail by Klopp [1], great uncertainties still arise as to the practical value of this form of therapy. Experimental and clinical knowledge, but also unanswered questions, will be discussed in the present chapter.

General Pharmacokinetic and Pharmacodynamic Aspects

For most cytostatics there exists a close correlation between toxicity and therapeutic efficacy [2]. Even if a cytostatic drug fails to affect tumour growth when given intravenously, it is quite possible that increased efficacy can be expected when the drug is given regionally. In addition to an increased concentration of the cytostatics in the tumour tissue, a lower total toxicity of the treatment is expected [3]. This effect occurs particularly in the regional chemotherapy of liver tumours, as the normal liver tissue may inactivate cytostatic substances before they pass into the whole organism (so-called first-pass effect). The dose limitation under these conditions is essentially a result of the metabolic performance of the healthy hepatic parenchyma. Exceeding the maximum tolerated dose by intraarterial administration may cause major systemic toxicity. The regional advantage of a single drug given by the intraarterial route depends largely on the extraction capacity of the liver [4]. Restrictions as to the advantage of a drug suggested by theoretical investigations therefore occur in the case of cirrhosis or advanced tumour involvement of the liver. Both conditions lead to a lower percentage of well-functioning liver parenchyma. Even the presence of arteriovenous shunts reduces the advantage of regional treatment. Interactions of different drugs administered simultaneously or sequentially within a short time interval (FAM, FUDRAM) probably would cause further limitations to regional drug delivery. Up to now no investigations on this topic have been reported.

The efficacy of regional cytostatic therapy is partly determined by the elimination of the drugs by the whole organism. Furthermore, the effect of regional drug administration also depends on the regional blood flow [4,5]. In the case of major arteriovenous shunts a higher systemic toxicity must be expected. Regional administration of a cytostatic will also offer less advantages if the therapeutic index of the drug is high after intravenous administration [6,7]. However, even regional therapy will remain ineffective as long as a tumour is resistant to high concentrations of the drug administered. As there are hardly any criteria yet enabling us to predict drug resistance, it remains open to what extent individual cytostatic tests of tumours can be of any value [8,9]. Of particular interest for regional chemotherapy of liver tumours are cytostatic substances that are metabolised primarily in the liver (high first-pass effect), having a short plasma half-life and a high whole-body clearance [3,4].

These requirements are fulfilled above all by the fluorinated pyrimidines (e.g., 5-FU, FUDR), which until now have most often been used in arterial infusion chemotherapy of the liver. Advantages in regional administration can also be expected for substances such as dichloromethotrexate, mitomycin C, and cisplatinum [3,10,11]. The whole body extraction rate, but also the first-pass effect in the liver, are affected by the quantity of substance administered, so that the selective advantage of regional administration of the drug can, possibly, be suspended dose-dependently. This may also be the case if two drugs are given at the same time, one affecting the extraction of the other. In this case, substances without a high primary clearance can become more effective than in the alternative intravenous injection only by means of primary higher flooding in the tumour cells. However, it cannot be generally assumed that, in the case of higher regional concentrations in a tumour-infested organ, the uptake in the tumour is greater than in normal tissue, since this also depends on the blood flow and vascularisation of the tumour tissue [12,13]. According to Ensminger and Gyves [3], the prerequisite for successful hepatic chemotherapy is to use the "correct" drug, which should have a degree of antitumour activity that may be expected to be improved by intraarterial administration. The dose-limiting toxicity should be extrahepatic and the pharmacokinetic properties should include a high total body clearance and a high extrahepatic clearance ratio (Table 1). Furthermore, a safe and reliable access to the tumour supplying arterial system with homogeneous distribution of the drug in the target organ is essential.

Questions to be answered are:

- Does intraarterial drug delivery yield increased tumour uptake of the cytostatic agent?
- Are combined chemotherapeutic treatment schedules such as FAM, CMF, FUDRAM advantageous if administered intraarterially?
- How do combined treatment schedules affect extraction ratios, systemic blood levels, and liver toxicity following intraarterial administration?

Table 1. Prerequisites for successful hepatic chemotherapy

A	Correct drug
	1. Appropriate degree of antitumour activity
	2. Dose-limiting toxicities should be extrahepatic
	3. Appropriate pharmacokinetic properties
	a) High total body clearance
	b) Hepatic extraction
	c) Extrahepatic clearance also present
B	Access to tumour blood supply complete and reliable
C	Reliable methods of administration
	1. External pumps
	2. Implantable devices

Studies Based on Animal Experiments

As the response to cytostatic therapy is multifactorial and partly unknown, it is difficult to assess the advantage of regional chemotherapy on the basis of clinical studies alone. Such studies compare different treatment methods, but important and possibly influencing parameters cannot be kept constant. Thus it is appropriate, despite all the problems of applicability, to make use of the results of standardised animal experiments. Most comparative studies on the efficacy of intraarterial and intravenous chemotherapy in various tumours in animal experiments demonstrate a superiority of regional therapy [14-17]. Obviously, it is the choice of cytostatic that plays a decisive role, but also the mode of administration affects the response rate. Animal experiments have demonstrated that, mostly for fluorinated pyrimidines, continuous long-term infusion therapy leads to better tumour regression than bolus injection [18]. Comparing intravenous and intraarterial bolus injections of FUDR with continuous infusion of the same drug, the tumour volume is 3-3.5 times larger after bolus treatment. In addition, there are fewer systemic side effects with continuous infusion than with short-term infusion. Until now this statement has been shown to be statistically significant only in animal experiments for 5-FU and FUDR [19]. Other results of interest show that, when comparing intraarterial and intraportal administration of the latter drug, the arterial chemotherapy is superior to the intraportal route [17]. The mean tumour volume in an Novikoff-hepatoma rat model was 3,400 ml after intraportal, 1,680 ml after intravenous, but only 680 ml after intraarteriaal administration of 1,220 µmol/kg FUDR continuously given for 5 consecutive days. According to our present knowledge, the advantage, at least for fluorinated pyrimidines, of intraarterial chemotherapy as opposed to other routes of administration (i.v. or intraportal) can be deduced from the results of animal experiments, provided it is performed as continuous treatment.

Clinical Experimental Studies

Studies with animal experiments can support the theoretical basis of a therapeutic concept, but the final documentation of the advantage of the treatment must be clinical. In addition to the experience of clinical studies, pharmacodynamic *in vitro* or *in vivo* studies are of particular interest here. The primary extraction and metabolism of cytostatics in the liver are responsible for the extent of systemic side effects. First of all it was appropriate to compare the cytostatic levels in the serum after intraarterial or intravenous systemic administration [3]. In this study the serum levels for fluorinated pyrimidines were found to be lower after intraarterial administration than after intravenous administration. This also explains the lower rate of side effects with regional administration than with systemic administration of fluorinated pyrimidines. Reduced plasma drug levels may also be attained by using microspheres together with the intraarterially given drug. This may improve the uptake of drugs with a low hepatic first-pass effect, e.g. adriamycin [20,21].

However, the tumour drug uptake is more decisive for the cytostatic effect of the therapy. This can be investigated by working up the biopsy material obtained during surgery [22,23]. These studies show that most patients display higher tumour tissue drug levels of radiolabelled cytostatics after intraarterial therapy and this further supports the concept of intraarterial regional therapy. While the drug uptake by the liver was identical after portal venous and intraarterial administration, the drug uptake by the tumour was 15 times higher following intraarterial than portal venous infusion. However, at present these studies permit no qualitative statement as to the subsequent cytostatic metabolism or anabolism in the tumour tissue. It is not the portion of the metabolised cytostatic that is decisive for the cytostatic efficacy, but the percent of cytostatically effective anabolites. Fluor^{19}-MR spectroscopy enables us to make a statement in this respect [24]. For this reason we are currently attempting, with the aid of this method, to obtain more accurate and more highly quantified statements [25]. The first results show that, in principle, it is possible to measure and differentiate metabolic and anabolic products in these probes during intraarterial or intravenous chemotherapy. But the percentage of cytotoxic anabolites, even after intraarterial administration, is extremely low and displays major individual fluctuations. Thus an advantage of intraarterial therapy cannot be assumed primarily in every individual patient [26]. Individualisation of the indications for treatment based on these examination techniques is therefore desirable for the future. Another way to study the uptake of pyrimidine antagonists is by means of positron emission tomography [27], which makes is possible to examine the tumour-to-tissue ratio under therapy *in vivo*. However, as long as such studies cannot be performed on a routine basis, one must deduce from the general clinical experience to what extent a treatment concept that may be brilliant in theory is actually confirmed and corroborated in clinical studies.

Questions to be answered are:

- To what extent does intraarterial drug administration increase the cytotoxic effect in cancer cells?
- Are there any specific criteria for liver malignancies, e.g., receptor proteins, microenvironmental factors, proportion of dormant cells, cell surface glycoproteins, that favour intraarterial drug uptake?

Initial Situation of Intraarterial Chemotherapy in Colorectal Liver Metastases

A statistically significant superiority of regional cytostatic chemotherapy in the treatment of colorectal liver metastases was shown only recently. There exists only one study in which regional cytostatic treatment of liver metastases was compared with an untreated control group from the point of view of survival [28]. By combining hepatic artery ligature and infusion chemotherapy of the portal vein with 5-FU, it was possible to achieve a slight prolongation of life. The significance of this study is, however, very limited due to the small number of cases it covers. A series of uncontrolled studies have also shown a higher response rate of the tumours after intraarterial therapy in comparison with intravenous treatment. A randomised study comparing short-term intraarterial and subsequent systemic 5-FU treatment with intravenous therapy alone was unable to show a significant difference [29]. However, owing to the very brief intraarterial treatment, the small number of patients, and an inadequate treatment technique, this study is subject to criticism. In these studies, treatment limitations were primarily due to the high risk of infection and thrombosis of the catheters which were inserted percutaneously [30]. As it is difficult to conduct controlled studies on regional chemotherapy with comparable patient groups, results from experimental animal studies are important [15,17]. Unfortunately, there are still no hard clinical data that prove the unrestricted advantage of continuous infusion chemotherapy compared to bolus or intermittent therapy with fluorinated pyrimidines. This may partly be explained by the fact that until a few years ago, it was practically impossible to give long-term, continuous chemotherapy in clinical studies.

Continuous Intraarterial Chemotherapy with FUDR in Colorectal Liver Metastases

The development of fully implantable drug delivery pumps created the possibility of practicable, continuous, regional cytostatic therapy. At present, however, their capacity and poor drug stability still limit their use and restrict it essentially to the administration of FUDR [31]. Additional bolus injection or short-term infusions may be performed by using the sideport of the pump model. Table 2 summarises some results of uncontrolled studies on intraarterial chemotherapy with FUDR using implantable pumps in patients with colorectal liver metastases. The considerable discrepancy between the published results is explained by the lack of uniform assessment criteria.

High response rates are mostly based on a drop in the CEA serum level by more than 30% as opposed to the initial value as the sole criterion [32-34]. As CEA varies due to circadian rhythms [35], the use of a drop in CEA as the sole response criterion is unacceptable. The response rates, which were obtained by means of imaging methods, are usually considerably lower (Table 2). Furthermore, in some subgroups of patients the course of CEA levels seems not to be of any significant prognostic value compared to imaging techniques.

Irrespective of this, the duration of the response to therapy would be more important but this information is missing in most publications. The decisive assessment criterion, however, remains the survival time of the patients treated intraarterially. One must take into consideration whether this is calculated from the time of the diagnosis of liver metastases or from the onset of intraarterial therapy. If one subjects these studies as much as possible to a comparable standard, the following picture emerges:

Calculated from the time of intraarterial catheter implantation, the median survival time of the patients is between 15 and 18 months. The tumour remission rate is about 40-50%, which is more than is generally expected following systemic chemotherapy. The median progression-free survival is 8 months. However, one should note that patients treated with the implantable pumps may represent a selected group. The selection criteria for these patients were in most studies a life expectancy of at least 3 months, a good general condition (Karnofsky Index >60), and no signs of hepatic insufficiency (bilirubin <2 mg/dl). In the study of Balch [32], 36% of

Table 2. Studies evaluating intraarterial FUDR chemotherapy using implantable pumps in colorectal liver metastases

Author	Patients	Response (%)				Survival (months) (median)	
		Imaging technique b)		CEA c)	Median duration (months)	Start of therapy	Time from diagnosis
		CR	PR				
Balch [32]	110	-	-	88 e)	-	-	24
Niederhuber [45]	93	-	76 a)	91	7	18	25
Shepard [34]	53	8	25	25	-	17	-
Rothmund [33]	22	32	32	77 e)	-	15	26
Chang [37]	20	5	57	60	7	16 d)	-
Hottenrott [46]	52	4	42	75 e)	>6	16	-
Kemeny [36]	45	2	48	60	11	15	-

a) Nuclide liver scan
b) CR + PR according to WHO criteria
c) More than 50% reduction
d) Calculated from date of randomisation
e) 30% reduction of CEA

the patients displayed no symptoms and had unilobar metastatic involvement of the liver, probably suitable for liver resection. This shows once again that nonrandomised, uncontrolled studies can lead to false conclusions.

Randomised Studies on Continuous Intraarterial Chemotherapy with FUDR

The need for randomised studies was not recognised until quite recently. Adequate final reports of the results of such studies have only been published by Kemeny and Chang [36,37] (Table 3). The total number of intraarterially treated patients in these two studies is only 65. The following can be deduced from the findings known to date:

The response rate for tumours treated with intraarterial chemotherapy is higher than after intravenous administration. However, the intraarterial FUDR dose was higher than the intravenous dose, due to toxicity problems [37]. Regardless of this, there is as yet no statistically significant effect on survival times in the two groups. It must be borne in mind that a crossover of the treatment with lack of response to the randomised therapy form was performed in most studies. Thus the actual treatment effect of one arm of therapy may be overlooked. On the other hand, it is clearly shown that, despite the better cytostatic response of liver metastases to intraarterial therapy, the survival time of the patients is determined by extrahepatic tumour progression. At present it is questionable to what extent this can be affected by combining intraarterial and intravenous therapy [34]. However, it is worth mentioning that, although systemic side effects can be reduced in intraarterial FUDR therapy, hepatobiliary local side effects are to be expected in a significant number of cases [38-42]. The most frequent regional side effect to be expected is chemical hepatitis (30-90% of all treated patients). Biliary sclerosis accompanying the treatment is considerably more severe. The rate of these severe side effects is dose-dependent and ranges between 5 and 56%. Biliary sclerosis may not only lead to discontinuation of the therapy but also to a shortening of the patient's survival time irrespective of the course of the disease [43].

Chemical hepatitis necessitates a reduction of the intraarterial FUDR dose of up to 40% [37]. Gastrointestinal side effects, such as gastroduodenitis and ulcers, were common in those studies that paid special attention to this feature (up to 50%) [43].

Table 3. Randomised trials evaluating intraarterial versus intravenous FUDR chemotherapy using implantable pumps in colorectal cancer

Author	Route of administration	No. Patients	Cross-over	Response (%)	Median survival (months)	Extrahepatic tumour progression (%)
Kemeny [36]	i.a.	45	+	51	15	43
	i.v.	49		22	15	15
Chang [37]	i.a.	20	-	62	16	50
	i.v.	29		17	13	20
Hohn [42]	i.a.	50	+	42	?	
	i.v.	64		9		
Hottenrott [46]	i.a.	26	-	52	16	54
	i.a. + i.v.	20		65	16	40

Continuous Intraarterial Chemotherapy with 5-FU

Considering the significant, mostly hepatobiliary side effects following continuous hepatic arterial infusion with FUDR, it is obvious that one should examine the possible advantages of other cytostatic drugs. Our experiences show that intraarterial chemotherapy with 5-FU produces favourable results, particularly as regards hepatobiliary toxicity [44]. On the other hand, the tumour remission rate is much lower with intraarterial 5-FU therapy than in most FUDR treatment series (Table 4). This difference may be of less importance, however, because the assessment of response rates may be based on different criteria. Another factor in favour of this is that the median survival time of the patients treated with 5-FU shows no difference compared to those treated with FUDR. The median progression-free period is also the same for both treatment regimens. Thus regional 5-FU chemotherapy has an advantage in that its toxicity is lower than that of FUDR treatment, while the efficacy is about the same. The advantage of regional 5-FU chemotherapy in colorectal liver metastases is supported further by the results of a recent study in which intraarterial 5-FU retreatment in patients who progressed under intravenous administration of the same drug was investigated [49]. A disadvantage is that continuous 5-FU therapy cannot be administered by means of implantable medication pumps; at present, reasonable doses can be administered only by means of external pumps. The technical complications here are greater and the patient is less comfortable during treatment [50,51].

Further Developments of Intraarterial Chemotherapy

Isolated perfusion of the liver is the most logical further development of an exclusively local cytostatic treatment method in which an attempt is made to administer a maximum dose of cytostatic to the tumour while avoiding systemic side effects [52]. Apart from requiring considerable surgical effort, the disadvantage of this procedure lies in the fact that the exposure to the cytostatics is only short and that, usually, the procedure cannot be repeated. Prolongation of the infusion time up to 4 hours resulted in 25% mortality [53]. Thus, the clinical findings of liver perfusion chemotherapy in primary and secondary liver tumours have also been disappointing so far [54]. In particular, the potential achievements

Table 4. Studies evaluating intraarterial long-term 5-FU chemotherapy in patients with colorectal liver metastases

					Side-Effects (%)			
Author	Patients (no.)	Drugs	Response (%)	Median survival (months)	Haemato-logic	Gastro-intestinal	Hepato-bilary	Technical problems
Denck [47]	50	6-7 g 5-FU for 3-6 d. q 6-8 w.	58	14		"minimal"		<5
Rougier [48]	43	1 g/m^2 BS for 6 h. weekly	56	>12[a]	18	9	-	65
Schlag [44]	33	1 g/m^2 BS for 5 d. q 3 w.	27	14	5	30	5	20

a Not specified, 79% of patients alive 12 months after onset of treatment

bear no relationship to the morbidity and mortality associated with the treatment.

In order to minimise hepatic and systemic toxicity reports on chronopharmacologic interactions between the circadian rhythm of plasma concentrations of cytostatic drugs, e.g., 5-FU, and drug-dependent toxicity should be taken into consideration [55].

Further developments of regional chemotherapy based on pharmacodynamic and tumourbiological considerations are more promising [4,21]. As the exposure of a tumour to cytostatics depends, among other things, on the intravasal hepatic blood flow, an increased concentration in the tumour tissue may be expected from a reduction of the flow rate. Therefore, attempts are being made to influence the blood flow in the hepatic artery by means of mechanical or pharmacological measures, in order to achieve greater efficacy and a broader therapeutic spectrum, including chemoembolisation, in which cytostatics are administered in mixtures with degradable starch microspheres, DSM [20], or Ethibloc®. Procedures in which cytostatics are administered directly incorporated into microsomes [56,57], or that utilise colloidal drug preparations [58], represent further developments of hepatic infusion chemotherapy that are worth pursuing.

Hyperthermia is a rather exciting treatment modality that may be applied in combination with intraarterial chemotherapy. The thermosensitivity of some types of cancer and a sensitising effect for drugs, e.g. bleomycin, give hope for further progress. Limiting problems will be the thermostability of cytostatic drugs and heating up of the whole liver parenchyma [59].

Final Assessment

Regional chemotherapy for primary and secondary liver cancer continues to be a theoretically attractive treatment concept although its clinical advantage has been proven only in some aspects. Thus it is a remarkable conclusion, after many years of clinical experience with this treatment form, that a large number of the studies performed are practically worthless since they do not permit a uniform assessment of the treatment results. For a long time the lack of a commonly accepted staging system for liver tumours made a comparison of intraarterial treatments versus others difficult or impossible, especially in the absence of untreated control groups. The side effects that are in some cases connected with this treatment and the usual lack of treatment effects on extrahepatic tumour growth by regional therapy are factors that should not be neglected. As it also remains unclear to what extent the survival time can be significantly prolonged with this treatment modality, one must also consider the patients' quality of life [51,60]. Some of the patients with untreated liver metastases display no symptoms for a long time. Thus it is difficult to know whether it is possible to improve the well-being of these patients by means of a treatment of uncertain efficacy but accompanied by side effects. On the other hand, we all know that with the current emphasis on active therapy it may be impossible to withhold any therapy option. This can considerably reduce a patient's optimism and thus his quality of life. The integration of regional chemotherapy into an overall therapy concept, as shown in Figure 1 for the treatment of colorectal liver metastases, is desirable. Under such conditions, the use of intraarterial chemotherapy seems to be worthwhile and appropriate.

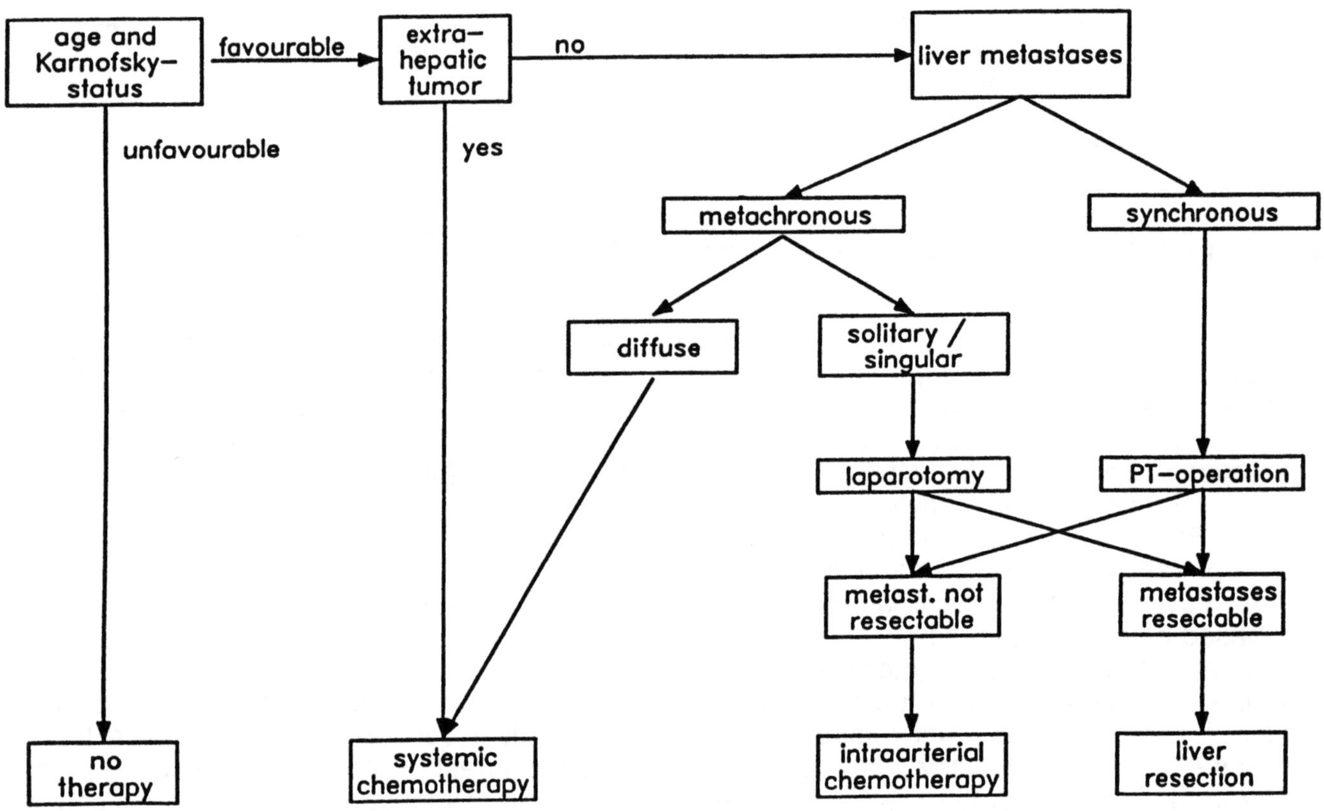

Fig. 1. Indication model in liver metastases of colorectal cancer (PT=primary tumour)

REFERENCES

1 Klopp CT, Alfrod TC, Bateman J, Berry GN, Whinship P: Fractionated intraarterial cancer chemotherapy with methyldiamine hydrochloride; preliminary report. Ann Surg (1950) 132:811-832

2 Frei E III, Canellos GP: Dose: a critical factor in cancer chemotherapy. Am J Med 1980 (69):585-594

3 Ensminger WD, Gyves JW: Regional Cancer chemotherapy. Cancer Treat Rep 1984 (68):101-115

4 Collins JM: Pharmacologic rationale for hepatic arterial therapy. In: Herfarth C, Schlag P, Hohenberger P (eds) Therapeutic Strategies in Primary and Metastatic Liver Cancer. Springer Verlag, Berlin Heidelberg New York Tokyo, 1986 pp 140-147

5 Chen H-SG, Gross JF: Intra-arterial infusion of anticancer drugs: theoretic aspects of drug delivery and review of responses. Cancer Treat Resp 1980 (64):31-40

6 Friedman MA: Systemic Therapies for Patients with Liver Tumors: Prospects for the Future. In: Herfarth C, Schlag P, Hohenberger P (eds) Therapeutic Strategies in Primary and Metastatic Liver Cancer. Springer Verlag, Berlin Heidelberg New York Tokyo, 1986 pp 112-113

7 Schreml W: Indications for treatment and determination of treatment effects with primary and secondary liver tumors. In: Herfarth Ch, Schlag P, Hohenberger P (eds) Therapeutic Strategies in Primary and Metastatic Liver Cancer. Springer Verlag, Berlin Heidelberg New York Tokyo, 1986 pp 91-102

8 Flentje D, Hohenberger P, Feichter G, Flentje M, Hess Ch, Schlag P: Kann das Ansprechen auf eine intraarterielle Chemotherapie bei Lebermetastasen colorectaler Carcinome vorhergesagt werden? Langenbecks Arch Chir 1986 (103 Suppl):331-336

9 Link KH, Aigner KR, Kühn W, Roetering N, Schwemmle K: Chemosensitivitätsbestimmung in vitro bei regionaler Chemotherapie von Lebertumoren. Tumor Diagnostik & Therapie 1985 (6):238-243

10 Kelsen DP, Hoffman J, Alcock N et al: Pharmacokinetics of regional infusion of cisplatin. Proc Am Assoc Cancer Res 1980 (21):745

11 Tseng MH, Luch J, Mittelman A, et al: Chemotherapy of advanced colorectal cancer with regional arterial mitomycin C infusion and concomitant measurement of serum drug level. Proc Am Assoc Cancer Res 1981 (22):359

12 Kaplan WD, Ensminger WD, Come SE, Smith EH, D'Orsi CJ, Levin DC, Takvorian RW, Steele GD Jr: Radionuclide angiography to predict patient response to hepatic artery chemotherapy. Cancer Treat Rep 1980 (64):1217-1222

13 Lehner B, Kretzschmar U, Bubeck B, Hölting T, Schlag P: Results of liver angiography and perfusion scintigraphy do not correlate with response to hepatic artery infusion chemotherapy. J Surg Oncol 1988 (39):73-78

14 Cotino H, Zwaveling A: Treatment of experimental liver tumors by continuous intra-arterial chemotherapy. Eur J Cancer 1976 (12):177-180

15 Bartkowski R, Berger MR, Aguiar JLA, Henne TH, Dörsam J, Geelhaar GH, Schlag P. Herfarth Ch: Experiments on the Efficacy and Toxicity of Locoregional Chemotherapy of Liver Tumors with 5-Fluoro-2'-Deoxyuridine (FUDR) and 5-Fluorouracil (5-FU) in an Animal Model. J Cancer Res Clin Oncol 1986 (111):42-46

16 Ridge JA, Collin C, Bading JR, Hancock C, Daly JM, Raaf JH: Regional infusion increases Adriamycin livels in hepatic implants of rabbit Vx-2 carcinoma. Cancer Res 1988 (48):4584-4587

17 Schlag P, Dörsam J, Aguiar JLA, Bartkowski R, Berger M: Hepatic arterial infusion (HAI) chemotherapy proves to be advantageous in the treatment of experimental liver tumors. Europ J Clin Oncol 1988 (24):1013-1018

18 Riemenschneider T, Ruf C, Späth G, Stuhldreier G, Elmouaouy A: Continuous or bolus chemotherapy with 5-fluoro-2'-deoxyuridine in transplanted experimental liver tumors? J Cancer Res Clin Oncol 1988 (114):482-486

19 Berger MR, Henne TH, Aguiar JLA, Bartowski R, Doersam J, Geelhaar GH, Schlag P, Herfarth Ch, Schmähl D: Experiments on the toxicity of locoregional liver chemotherapy with 5-fluoro2'-deoxyuridine and 5-fluorouracil in an animal model. In: Herfarth Ch, Schlag P, Hohenberger P (eds) Therapeutic Strategies in Primary and Metastatic Liver Cancer (RRCR Vol 100). Springer Verlag, Berlin Heidelberg New York Tokyo 1986 pp 148-156

20 Lindell B, Aronsen K, Nosslin B, Rothman U: Studies in pharmacokinetics and tolerance of substances temporarily retained in the liver by microsphere embolisation. Ann Surg 1978 (187):95-99

21 Sigurdson ER, Ridge JA, Daly JM: Intra-arterial infusion of doxorubicin with degradable starch microspheres: Improvement of hepatic tumor drug uptake. Arch Surg 1986 (121):1277-1281

22 Ridge JA, Sigurdson ER, Daly JM: Distribution of fluorodeoxyuridine (FUdR) uptake in human liver and colorectal hepatic metastases after arterial infusion. Surg Gynecol Obstet 1987 (164):319-323

23 Sigurdson ER, Ridge JA, Kemeny N, Daly JM: Tumor and liver drug uptake following hepatic artery and portal vein infusion. J Clin Oncol 1987 (5):1836-1840

24 Malet-Martino MC, Faure F, Vialaneix JP, Palevody C, Hollande E, Martino R: Noninvasive fluorine-19 NMR study of fluoropyrimidine metabolism in cell cultures of human pancreatic and colon adenocarcinoma. Cancer Chemother Pharmacol 1986 (18):5-10

25 Semmler W, Bachert-Baumann P, Gückel F, Lehner B, Schlag P, van Kaick G: Non invasive monitoring of the 5-Fluorouracil catabolism and anabolism in patients by means of 19F MRS: Comparison of intraarterial and intravenous administration. 7th Annual Meeting of the Society of Magnetic Resonance in Medicine. San Francisco 1988 (1):258

26 Daly JM, Butlerm J, Kemeny N. Yeh SDJ, Ridge JA, Botet J, Bading JR, DeCosse JJ, Benua RS: Predicting Tumor Response in Patients with Colorectal Hepatic Metastases. Ann Surg 1985 (202):384-393

27 Abe Y, Fukuda H, Ishiwata K, Yoshioka S, Yamada K, Endo S, Kubota K, Sato T, Matsuzawa T,

Takahashi T, Ido T: Studies on 18F-labelled pyrimidines, tumor uptakes of 18F-5-fluorouracil, 18F-5-fluorouridine and 18F-5-fluorodeoxyuridine in animals. Eur J Nucl Med 1983 (8):258-261
28 Taylor I: Cytotoxic perfusion for colorectal liver metastases. Br J Surg 1978 (65):219-222
29 Grage TB, Vassilopoulos PP, Shingleton WW, Jubert AV, Moss SE: Results of a prospective randomized study of hepatic artery infusion with 5-fluorouracil vs intravenous 5-fluorouracil in patients with hepatic metastases from colorectal cancer: a Central Oncology Group Study. Surgery 1979 (86):550-555
30 Reed ML, Vaitkevicius K, Al-Sarraf M, Vaughn PC, Ainghakowinta A, Sexon-Porte M, Izbick R, Baker L, Straatsma GW: The practicability of chronic hepatic artery infusion therapy of primary and metastatic hepatic malignancies; ten year results of 124 patients in a prospective trial. Cancer 1981 (42):402
31 Schlag P: Continuous cancer chemotherapy - rationale and prerequisites for treatment at home. Int J Tech Ass Health Care 1985 (1):18-20
32 Balch CM, Urist MM, McGregor ML: Continuous regional chemotherapy for metastatic colorectal cancer using a totally implantable infusion pump. Am J Surg 1983 (145): 285-290
33 Rothmund M, Brückner R, Keller E, Quint B, Knuth A, Schicketanz K: Chemotherapie bei Lebermetastasen colorectaler Carcinome mit implantierbaren Gasdruckpumpen - Ergebnisse einer prospektiven Studie. Dtsch Med Wschr 1986 (111):652-658
34 Hottenrott C, Lorenz M: Stellenwert der regionalen Chemotherapie der Leber. Z Gastroenterologie 1987 (25):364-373
35 Focan C, Focan-Henrad D, Collette J, Mechkouri M, Levi F, Hrushesky W, Touitou Y, Franchimont P: Cancer-associated alteration of circadian rhythm in carcinoembryonic antigen (CEA) and alpha-fetoprotein (AFP) in humans. Anticancer Res 1986 (6):1137-1144
36 Kemeny N, Daly J, Reichman B, Geller N, Botet J, Oderman P: Intrahepatic systemic infusion of fluorodeoxyuridine (FUDR) in patients with liver metastases from colorectal carcinoma. Ann Int Med 1987 (107):459-465
37 Chang AE, Schneider PD, Sugarbaker PH, Simpson C, Culnane M, Steinberg SM: A Prospective Randomized Trial of Regional Versus Systemic Continuous 5-Fluorodeoxyuridine Chemotherapy in the Treatment of Colorectal Liver Metastases. Ann. Surg 1987 (206):685-693
38 Kemeny N, Daly J, Oderman P, Shike M, Chun H, Petroni G, Geller N: Hepatic artery pump infusion: toxicity and results in patients with metastatic colorectal carcinoma. J Clin Oncol 1984 (2): 595-600
39 Shepard KV, Levin B, Karl RC et al: Therapy for metastatic colorectal cancer with hepatic artery infusion chemotherapy using a subcutaneous implanted pump. J Clin Oncol 1985 (3):161-169
40 Johnson LP, Rivkin SE: The implanted pump in metastatic colorectal cancer of the liver - risk versus benefit. Am J Surg 1985 (149):595-598
41 Kemeny M, Goldberg D, Beatty JD, Blayney D, Browning S, Doroshow J, Ganteaume L, Hill RL, Kokal WA, Riihimaki DU, Terz JJ: Results of a prospective randomized trial of continuous regional chemotherapy and hepatic resection as treatment of hepatic metastases from colorectal cancer. Cancer 1986 (57):492-498
42 Hohn D, Stagg R, Rayner A, Lewis B: The NCOG randomized trial of intravenous (IV) vs hepatic arterial (IA) FUDR for colorectal cancer metastatic to the liver. III Intern Conference on Advances in Regional Cancer Therapy 1987: Abstract B6
43 Hohn DC, Rayner AA, Economou JS, Ignoffo RJ, Lewis BJ, Stagg RJ: Toxicities and complications of implanted pump hepatic arterial and intravenous floxuridine infusion. Cancer 1986 (57):465-470
44 Schlag P, Hohenberger P, Schwarz V, Herfarth C: Intraarterielle 5-Fluorouracil-Chemotherapie bei Lebermetastasen colorectaler Carcinome. Med Klinik 1988 (83):705-709
45 Niederhuber E, Ensminger WD, Gyves J, Thrall J, Walker S, Cozzi E: Regional chemotherapy of colorectal cancer metastatic to the liver. Cancer 1984 (53):1336-1343
46 Hottenrott C, Lorenz M, Encke A: Kann der Erfolg einer lokalen Chemotherapie der Leber durch eine zusätzliche systemische Zytostase verbessert werden ? Eine randomisierte Multicenterstudie. Langenbecks Archiv Chir 1987 (Abstr 262)
47 Denck H: Ergebnisse einer intraarteriellen intermittierenden Chemotherapie mit 5-FU bei Metastasenleber sowie inoperablen Tumoren des Gastrointestinal- und Urogenitaltraktes. Onkologie 1984 (7):167-176
48 Rougier Ph, Laser Ph, Elias D, Ghosn M, Droz JP, Sidibe S, Theodore C, Lumbroso J: Intraarterial hepatic chemotherapy (IAHC) for liver metastasis (LM) from colorectal (CR) origin. Proc ASCO 1987 (6): Abstr 369
49 Hohenberger P, Schlag P, Raeth U, Herrmann R: Progressive liver metastases of colorectal cancer after systemic chemotherapy - Results of intrahepatic retreatment using fluoropyrimidines. Am J Clin Oncol 1989 (accepted for publication)
50 Civalleri D, Cafiero F, Cosimelli M, Craus W, Doci R, Repetto M, Simoni G: Regional arterial chemotherapy of liver tumours. I. Performance comparison between a totally implantable pump and a conventional access system. Eur J Surg Oncol 1986 (12):277-282
51 Schlag P, Feil H, Ruoff G, Hohenberger P, Hölting T, Buhl K: Onkologische Behandlung zu Hause: Erfahrungen mit einer ambulanten intraarteriellen Chemotherapie von Lebermetastasen. Schweiz Med Wschr 1987 (117):1342-1346
52 Sindelar WF: Isolation-Perfusion of the Liver with 5-Fluorouracil. Ann Surg 1985 (201):337-343
53 Skibba JL, Quebbeman EJ: Tumoricidal effects and patient survival after hyperthermic liver perfusion. Arch Surg 1986 (121):1266-1271
54 Schwemmle K, Aigner K: Requirements and results of liver perfusion. In: Herfarth Ch, Schlag P, Hohenberger P (eds) Therapeutic Strategies in Primary and Metastatic Liver Cancer. Springer Verlag, Berlin Heidelberg New York Tokyo, 1986 pp 229-233
55 Petit E, Milano G, Levi F, Thyss A, Bailleul F, Schneider M: Circadian rhythm-varying plasma

concentration of 5-fluorouracil during a five-day continuous venous infusion at a constant rate in cancer patients. Cancer Res 1988 (48):1676-1679
56 Kato T, Nemoto R, Mori H, Kumagai I: Sustained-release properties of microencapsulated mitomycin C with ethylcellulose infused into the renal artery of the dog. Cancer 1980 (46):14-21
57 Gabizon A, Goren D, Fuks Z, Barenholz Y, Dagan A, Meshorer A: Enhancement of adriamycin delivery to liver metastatic cells with increased tumoricidal effect using liposomes as drug carriers. Cancer Res 1983 (43):4730-4735
58 Bachur NR, Friedman RD, Hollenbeck RG: Physicochemical characteristics of ferric adriamycin complexes. Cancer Chemother Pharmacol 1984 (12):5-9
59 Issels RD, Wilmanns W: Application of hyperthermia in the treatment of cancer. In: Recent Results in Cancer Research, Vol 108. Springer Verlag, Berlin, Heidelberg, New York, Tokyo 1988
60 Sugarbaker PH et al: Quality of life and cost effectiveness issues in the management of patients with hepatic metastases from colorectal cancer. In: Mastromarino A (ed): Biology and Treatment of Colorectal Cancer Metastasis. M Nijhoff, Boston 1984 pp 83-100

Chemoembolisation in Regional Chemotherapy

H.P.J.M. Noteborn and J.G. McVie

Department of Experimental Therapy, The Netherlands Cancer Institute, Amsterdam, The Netherlands

Introduction

Metastases from primary gastrointestinal cancers to the liver contribute to the morbidity and mortality of up to 25% of all cancer patients. The prognosis of patients with liver metastases from a primary tumour in colon or rectum is poor, i.e., 70% of them will die within one year and at two years only 8-10% remain alive [1]. Surgical resection is the only current means of achieving a cure for unilobar liver colorectal metastases resulting in survival times of more than 5 years. Despite recent advances in early diagnosis and general patient care, less than 5% of all cases of colorectal cancer metastatic to liver and about 10% of all primary hepatocellular carcinomas are truly resectable for cure [1-4]. As extensive trials with systemic chemotherapy and hepatic arterial occlusion, either by ligation or by embolisation, have yielded disappointing response rates, the treatment of liver metastases still constitutes a major oncologic challenge [5,6].

This chapter reviews the state of the art of chemoembolisation in regional therapy with particular reference to liver-only involvement, when liver metastasis is the main disease to be treated. An attempt will be made to provide an insight into theoretical aspects, as well as the particular applications of delivery systems that utilise properties of microparticulate (15-200 microns) devices and drug-oil suspensions to achieve transient or persistent chemoembolisation in the first capillary bed encountered.

Therapeutic and toxic effects of chemotherapeutic agents are related to the time the active principal is exposed in an effective concentration to its target. The therapeutic index of drugs may therefore be improved by modifying the delivery schedule to expand the dwell time, in order to increase the exposure of the growth fraction of tumour tissue to the drug. So far, the results of continuous or prolonged systemic cytostatic treatment in metastatic colorectal cancer have been disappointing. No single agent or combination drug programme can be considered standard. Limits are the relative resistance of solid tumours and systemic side effects. Frequently, 5-fluorouracil (5-FU) is used as a single agent and, depending upon dose and mode of administration, it results in a response rate of approximately 15-30% [6]. Its effect on median survival, however, is minimal [7-9], but in terms of palliation the frequency of severe and life-threatening toxicity was significantly less for long-term infusion schedules [6,10-17].

On the other hand, the narrow therapeutic index of most anticancer drugs has increased clinical interest in regional infusion schedules, and hepatic arterial infusion (HAI) in particular. HAI is designed to deliver high drug concentrations to a limited area and, simultaneously (depending on the type of drug) a significant amount of drug will be fractionally extracted during first pass through the capillary bed of the target region resulting in lower systemic drug exposure [18-21]. Although recent developments have made HAI a more rational therapy, the clinical response rates only justify the use of 5-fluoro-2'-deoxyuridine (FUDR) [6,22-25]. However, the potential for long-term survival seems to exist only in those patients with resectable liver neoplasms; for all others, palliation and an overall benefit on quality of life is the best result that can be expected [2,6,11,26-30].

fusion via the hepatic artery still offers a theoretical advantage by selective targeting of drugs into tumour vessels derived from preexisting arterial branches [31].

What Are the Possibilities for Pharmacologic Improvement of Hepatic Arterial Infusion?

Current chemotherapy of liver metastases probably does not adequately restrict the disposition of anticancer drugs within tumours, but usually causes still too much concomitant cytotoxicity to normal tissue of the host. In recognition of this problem, various strategies have been developed to improve clinical results with conventional cytotoxic anticancer therapy. These include the combination of drugs to prevent the occurence of drug resistance, the development of agents with more tumour-specific effects, the delivery of drugs by vascular access to specific organs and directly to tumours within them.

Collins [32] and Ensminger and Gyves [33] defined the rationale in determining whether an anticancer drug is pharmacologically suitable for regional arterial therapy against, for example, liver metastases. Supposing that both cancer cell kill and toxicity to normal tissue are linearly proportional to exposure of the drug (C x T), the relative efficacy (Ref) of intra-arterial as opposed to intravenous routes may be defined by equation 1 [22]:

$$\text{(1)}\quad \text{Ref} = 1 + \frac{\text{(apparent plasma clearance)}}{\text{(tumour plasma flow)}}$$

In contrast, the relative advantage in the reduction of systemic toxicity (Rtox) is solely a function of the extraction ratio (ER) of the drug by the infused area (or tumour) as described by equation 2 [22]:

$$\text{(2)}\quad \text{Rtox} = \frac{1}{(1 - \text{ER})}$$

Thus, the ratio of total body clearance of a drug to its regional exchange rate or blood flow is the principal determinant of therapeutic advantage by regional chemotherapy [22,32]. Based on this linear pharmacokinetic model, the most favorable circumstances for locoregional drug delivery are as listed in Table 1.

Table 1. Parameters of importance for regional drug delivery

1)	cytotoxic agents with a high total body clearance
2)	steep dose-response for the tumour in question
3)	significant activity in that tumour type
4)	high hepatic extraction and/or metabolism of the drug
5)	sites of delivery with low blood exchange rates

Equations (1) and (2) [22] indicate that from the point of view of both the tumour and systemic circulation there is only a limited pharmacologic advantage for regional chemotherapy into organs with plasma flows in excess of 350 ml/m^2 per min (human liver [34]), except when tumour plasma flows are low or blocked. To achieve this last goal, drugs are often coupled to carriers; e.g., macromolecules (antibodies, glycoproteins, polymers), cellular vectors (red blood cell ghosts, platelets) and colloidal carriers (emulsions, liposomes, nanoparticles, microspheres, microcapsules).

One clear rationale for site-directed and locally targeted chemotherapy of drugs attached to carriers is to protect the drug from the *in-vivo* environment during transport until subsequent release at the target site. Another comprehensive goal of occlusion cancer chemotherapy is to reduce the tumour-host imbalance by altering the distribution, uptake and efficacy of cytotoxic agents in such a way that effective cytotoxicity is obtained in malignant cells only. Ideally, after prompt release of drug from the carrier, the carrier should be eliminated without any severe foreign body toxicity.

Blood Supply of Liver Metastasis

The blood supply of metastases is of great importance, because numerous innovative drug delivery techniques are essentially dependent on tumour vascularity. Despite rapid progress in the knowledge on the vascular morphology of liver metastases [5,35-37], there is still a lack of quantitative data on the rheological properties of blood and microvascular pressures in tumour circulation (for a review see ref. 38). Whereas in systemic chemotherapy blood flow plays an important role in the delivery of cytostatics, the efficacy of carrier-mediated loco-regional treatment of hepatic cancers depends almost exclusively upon the local blood flow and vascular morphology.

The tumour vasculature is highly heterogeneous, and is determined to some extent by the growth pattern of cancer cells. Continuous studies on the macroscopic organisation of experimental tumours implanted into the liver of rodents [5,31] have demonstrated that the hepatic tumour vasculature is primarily that of an encircling plexus of vessels at the periphery of the tumour. Moreover, the vasculature of small-sized hepatic lesions (less than 2 mm in diameter) is derived for 70-90% from portal venules [5,35,38]. In larger tumours (more than 0.3 g in weight) the encircling vessels are filled predominantly by arterial circulation (up to 95%) [5,31,35], are often well-developed and hypervascularity is dominant. Central portions of experimental tumours are usually relatively hypovascular (haemorrhagic necrosis). When these tumours grow to a very large size (up to 35 mm in diameter), vascularity seems to be split up into arterial and portal, and into hypervascular and avascular [5].

In humans, there are no quantitative data on the macroscopic vascular morphology of metastatic tumours. So far, only hepatic angiography appears to be a useful diagnostic tool in determining the degree of vascularity in different tumour types. In general, primary hepatomas tend to be more vascular than metastases of carcinoid tumours, islet cell carcinomas, sarcomas, and renal cell carcinomas. Tumours of breast, colon, pancreas, and endometrium are only moderately vascular; metastases from squamous cell carcinomas of the lung, adenocarcinomas of stomach, pancreas and breast, and melanomas are often avascular [4,5]. As yet, there are no quantitative data in the literature available on the detailed branching pattern of these vessels in human tumours [4,5,35-37 and ref. 38 for details].

Similarly, quantitative data on blood flow in liver metastases are of utmost importance for the accessibility of local targeting therapy attached to carriers. This approach depends upon: 1) the homogeneous distribution throughout the liver of carriers without shunting to the venous circulation (e.g., 15 micron microspheres [51]), 2) differentially greater arterial blood supply to hepatic tumours as opposed to normal liver parenchyma (e.g., tumour-liver ratios in the order of 2.4 to 4.8 [31,35]), 3) blood viscosity and geometric resistance for a network of vessels, and 4) drops in arteriolar-venular pressure gradients [38]. On the other hand, portal venous flow to hepatic metastases has consistently been demonstrated as less than for normal liver tissue [5,30,39]. In humans, using arterial infusion of 99m-Tc labelled macroaggregated albumin, it could be shown that in 18 patients (26 lesions) the uptake of colloidal material into tumour tissue compared with healthy areas of the liver varied from 1.2 to 8.0 (median 2.7) [36,40,41]. Studies in our laboratory using 99m-Tc labelled albumin microspheres (15-35 microns in diameter) injected into the hepatic artery circulation were performed in 5 patients with metastatic hepatic tumours [41]. An up to 10-fold increase of sphere-uptake was noted in the tumour deposits. These findings are ascribed to an extra capillary network in about 80% of all liver metastases, which causes the blockage of microspheres [31,42,43] (Fig. 1). This phenomenon most likely forms the basis for the use of colloidal suspensions for intra-arterial regional chemotherapy of human liver metastases [42-45]. In addition, arterio-venous shunting has been found to increase when the capillary flow is blocked by starch microspheres [53]. Degradable starch microspheres (DSM or Spherex) might therefore have an additional value in diverting the blood flow to the hypovascular areas after occlusion of well-vascularised parts in hepatic tumours [44].

Since the deposition of these vascular tracers in liver is cumulative due to capillary occlusion, these techniques may not supply definitive information about the haemodynamics of liver metastases [36,38,46]. Arterial blood flow in hepatic cancers has therefore been studied with radionuclide flow methods [36,46]. Sasaki et al. [36] reported tumour/non-tumour

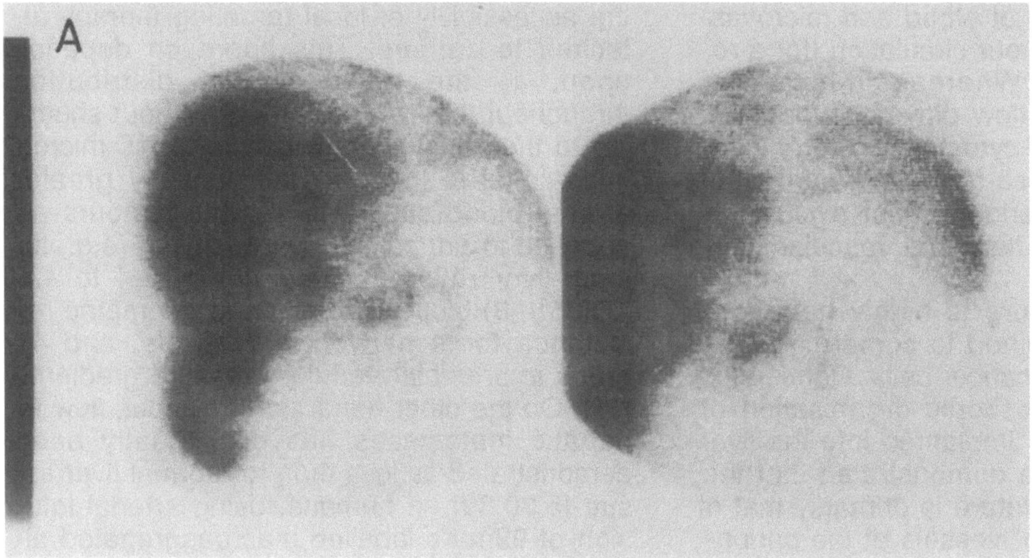

Fig. 1. (A) Liver imaging with intravenously administered [99m-Tc] Sn colloid of a patient (female, 52 years old) with liver cell carcinoma delineating normal functional liver tissue whilst leaving non-functional tumour tissue as a cold spot

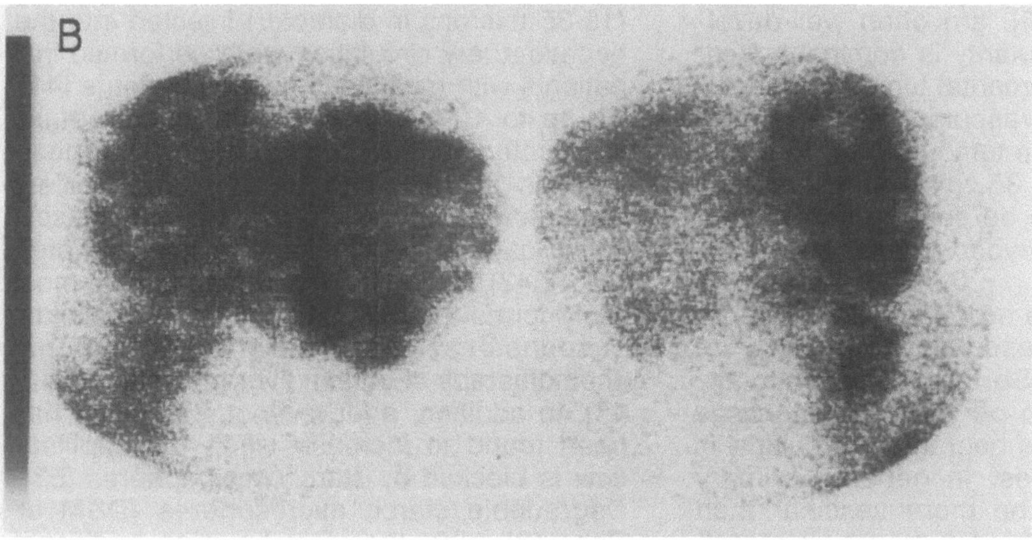

(B) [99m-Tc] microsphere scan of same patient after intra-arterial hepatic albumin microsphere (15-35 microns in diameter) infusion. Note site-directed delivery of microspheres to tumour lesions with lower accumulation in normal liver parenchyma

ratios of the arterial flow between 1.03 to 3.69 (median 2.11) studying 13 patients with hepatocellular carcinoma (32 lesions), but these authors noted that the arterial blood flow to tumours was effected by the patients position [36]. Merkel et al. [46] evaluated the blood flow of experimental mature liver metastases in rat by locally injected 133-Xenon washout. Considering the tumour mass as a whole, it was concluded that Walker-256 hepatic carcinomas show hypoperfusion or a relatively stagnant blood flow/unit mass as tumour size increases. In contrast to these findings, experiments on salivary adenocarcinoma in the liver of rats in which arterial blood flow was calculated after injection of cobalt-57 microspheres (15 micron in diameter) demonstrated that, regardless of tumour size studied, the blood flow/unit mass at the periphery of the lesion remained constant [31].

It is difficult to make a direct comparison of these animal experiments [31,46], but for therapeutic purposes this has significance in that flow to the periphery might be increased but flow to the central areas markedly decreased. These results may also be indicative of the development of collateral flow. Obviously, understanding the precise relationship between vascularity and functional flow, together with the role of blood rheology and geometric resistance for a network of vessels in tumours, would help in modifying blood flow and transport of cytostatics in hepatic lesions.

Site-Directed and Local Targeting of Drugs by Chemoembolisation

Knowledge concerning angiogenesis, vascularity and blood flow of hepatic metastases and pharmacokinetics of several infusion systems has led to the development of potential microparticulate carriers aimed at selectively attacking the tumour by utilising circulatory differences [31,42]. Chemoembolisation refers to the intraarterial coadministration of drugs and vascular occlusive devices to treat cancer. The suggestion here is that introduction of anticancer drug carrying particles of requisite size into the arterial system of, e.g., metastatic liver cancer, either causes tumour infarction by occlusion or induces transient ischaemia within the tumour microvasculature, whereupon the vascular entrapped drug can be released locally as the particulate carrier slowly biodegrades. Moreover, tissue permeability is increased due to anoxia, allowing the drug to permeate into the tissue more easily. The portal blood flow supports hepatocytes during ischaemia and clears drug from these cells but not from areas with tumour lesions. This approach has been utilised successfully with: 1) biodegradable microspheres manufactured from albumin [47-52], starch (DSM or Spherex) [53-57], ethylcellulose [58,59] or polylactic acid [60-68] as matrix material; 2) nanoparticles from alkylcyanoacrylate [69-73]; and 3) lipiodol emulsions [74-77].

Colloidal Drug Carriers: Controlled Release Devices for Parenteral Application and Transient or Persistent Blocking Agents for Tumour Vasculature

Colloidal carriers consist of spherical networks of polymers entrapping a drug inside or throughout the matrix with the potential for controlled release of the active molecule from the system after re-hydration. The maximum amount of drug incorporated into the carrier prepared either using fixation, solvent vaporation, phase extraction or polymerisation emulsion processes with drug dissolved in the (non)aqueous phase is dependent on the liquid/liquid distribution coefficient and the extent of polymer binding. The following definitions are usually used: Particles with diameters less than 1.0 micron are called nanoparticles, and those with a mean particle diameter of 1.0 micron or more are designated as microspheres. The difference between microspheres and microcapsules depends on the fact that the latter have solid envelopes containing the active molecule inside its core, whereas microspheres consist of continuous matrices with uniformly dispersed drug.

Passive and Active Targeting Using Colloidal Carrier-Associated Drugs

Widder et al. [80] described the carrier-mediated targeting of drugs to their sites of action as a multi-order event, first order being the specific distribution of the colloidal carrier over a particular organ (including endothelial passage), second order being the selective targeting only to diseased parts of the organ, and third order being the selective intracellular delivery. Figure 2 illustrates the rationales for the use of microparticulate material as targetable drug devices.

Radiolabelled microspheres of various sizes and composition have been used extensively for lung scans and circulatory studies (for a review see ref. 82). In general, the partitioning

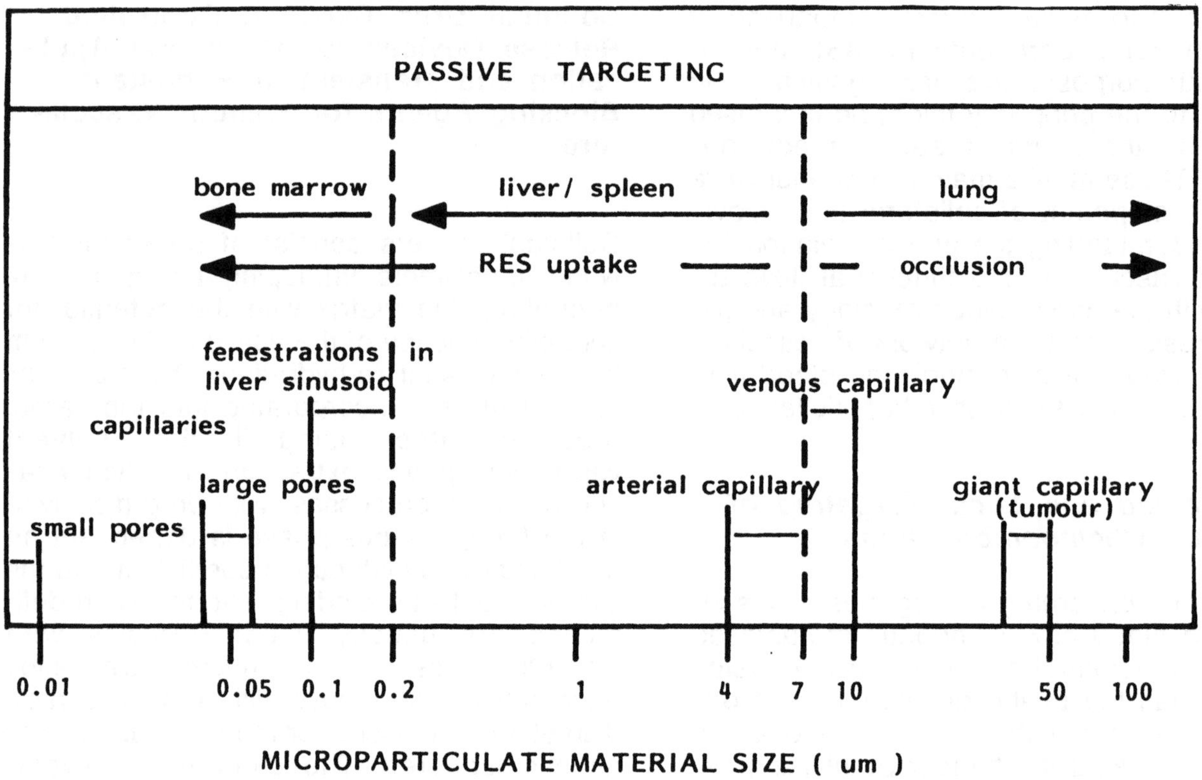

Fig. 2. The vascular bed and passive targeting of delivered microparticulate suspensions. Modified from ref. [43,78,79]

of colloidal suspensions in the body depends primarily upon their sizes (passive targeting), which can be distinguished by 3 patterns [43,78]:

- intravenous, intra-arterial or intraperitoneal injection of non-agglomerated particles smaller than 4.0 microns tend to be rapidly cleared from the general circulation by macrophages of the RES, and localised in Kupffer cells of the liver;
- intravenous injection of particles above 7 to 12 microns leads to their mechanical filtration by the lungs; particles between 3 to 12 microns have the capacity to lodge in the capillary beds of lung, liver, spleen and tumours;
- regional intra-arterial delivery of colloidal particles larger than 12 micron are completely trapped by transient or persistent capillary blockage.

The partitioning of microspheres within a target circulation is proportional to the local blood flow [36,40], which may result in a homogeneous capillary distribution. Second-order targeting [5,27,31,41,42] of colloidal carriers can be obtained by altering their shape and surface characteristics [71]. In particular, the adsorption of plasma components (immuno-opsonins, fibronectin, platelets and fibrin) onto the surface remains a rather unpredictable factor. Many studies are therefore directed towards approaches to divert nanoparticles from the RES, and include coating of the surface [82-84], the incorporation of small magnetic particles in spheres, hence permitting site-specific delivery with the use of extracorporeal two-dimensional magnetic fields [80,85], or saturation of RES uptake by injection of large doses of empty colloidal particles [51,62,71]. This latter approach, however, may be dangerous since the immune system will be compromised [86], and the phagocytotic activity of the RES may be altered by neoplastic diseases [87].

Selective tumour targeting without systemic toxicity has been demonstrated in Yoshida sarcoma-bearing rats using biodegradable magnetic microspheres of 1.0 microns in diameter entrapping doxorubicin [80]. Single-dose therapy with these doxorubicin-magnetite spheres resulted in complete remission in 77% and in significant regression in 13% of the animals, while the same drug dose was ineffective in controls. The exact potential and limitations of magnetic microspheres still have to be assessed in human tumours. One of the main problems arising when magnetically guided spheres are used is its limited use to body parts like extremities and tumours localised near the surface of the body [88]. The neutrophil chemo-attractant N-formyl-methionylleucyl-phenylalanine (f-MLP) has been encapsulated in magnetite microspheres (0.6 microns in diameter) [89]. This tetrapeptide is extremely toxic and even lethal in freely circulating form. However, site-specific delivery of about 40% of the spheres to the thoracic viscera by magnetic targeting showed that all bioactive f-MLP was released within 0 to 24 hours, giving high local levels in the right lung of the rat with free plasma levels of f-MLP remaining at all times below critical levels by a factor 100 [89]. These examples of incorporating a drug into biodegradable carriers followed by site-specific delivery demonstrated clearly that, firstly, it minimises systemic toxicity remarkably; secondly, it achieves high local drug concentrations and, thirdly, the entrapping procedure does not affect the *in vivo* biological activity of an anticancer drug. This system therefore meets the defined rationales for pharmacologically designed drug delivery [18,19,28,29].

Uptake mechanisms from the extravascular space into the intracellular space of tumour cells are different compared with normal cells. From the analysis by Ackerman [5] of the vascular permeability of liver tumours, it follows that reactive hyperaemia, damage to the endothelial lining of vessels, and vascular stasis causes an increased vascular permeability in hepatocellular carcinoma compared with that of host tissue. Since they are particulate, microspheres can be actively internalised by tumour cell lines that exhibit enhanced endocytotic and lysosomotropic actvities [90,91]. Albumin nanoparticles containing mercaptopurine are phagocytised *in vitro* by HeLa, KB and human glioblastoma cells [69]. Lewis Lung carcinoma cells are able to accumulate *in vivo* nanoparticles [92]. Moreover, we observed that even albumin microspheres 15-25 microns in diameter are accumulated *in vitro* by B16 melanoma cells (Fig. 3).

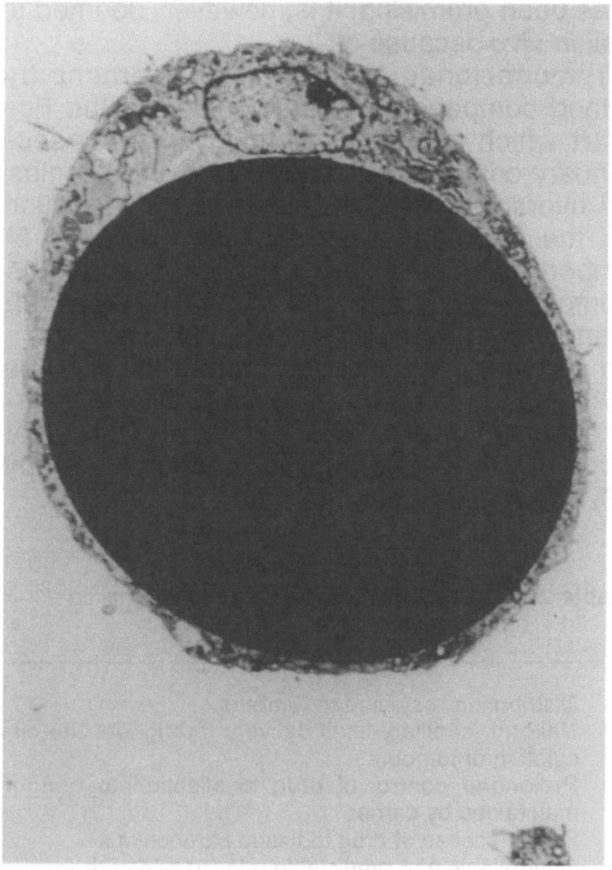

Fig. 3. *In vitro* phagocytosis of 15-25 micron human albumin microspheres by a B16 murine melanoma tumour cell (x 3500)

The fraction of incorporated drug that is delivered to the intracellular compartments depends upon both the rate of drug release and the rate of phagocytic uptake of the carrier. Inflammatory processes at the tumour site lead to structural changes of capillaries, which may facilitate the passage of carriers through the endothelial wall. Third-order targeting is possible using nanoparticles, although this is minimised by employing carriers of intermediate stability that afford rapid release at predominantly extracellular sites. Actually, some recent evidence suggests that tumour cells integrate into linings of blood vessels [93], and that there is contact possible between drug-loaded spheres and these tumour cells [94].

Another approach to the introduction of targeted chemotherapy is the reaction of colloidal carriers with the Fc-portion of tumour-specific antibodies [73,95,96]. *In vitro* tumour vectoring of antibody-microsphere conjugates

has been promising; it is, however, doomed to fail *in vivo* because of:
1) monoclonal antibody displacement by blood components, 2) recognition of the Fc-part which stimulates phagocytosis, 3) secondary coating due to adsorption of opsonins, 4) oversized particles that enable penetration of the endothelial wall of blood vessels, 5) impermeability of the endothelium near the tumour, and 6) antigens originating from the xenograft in liver and spleen [90,91].
In summary, drug-loaded carriers have to be designed in such a way as to fulfil both pharmaceutical and biological criteria of an ideal drug delivery system for loco-regional therapy [6,12,17-19,27-29,42] (Table 2).

Table 2. Requirements for the ideal drug carrier in regional therapy

1) Distribution restricted to tumours
2) Uniform, capillary-level delivery throughout the circulation of tumours
3) Prolonged control of drug localisation to tumour maintained by carrier
4) Ready access of drug to tissue parenchyma
5) Controllable and predictable release rate of drug
6) Carrier device for a wide spectrum of commercially available drugs
7) Biocompatible surface properties and non-immunogenic
8) Biodegradable and non-toxic catabolic products

At this point, we consider that biodegradable microspheres manufactured from albumin, starch, gelatin, acryloylated polysaccharides or polylactic acid as matrix polymers for the formulation of cytostatic agents afford a much greater probability than ethylcellulose, isobutyl 2-cyanoacrylate or polystyrene-spheres in providing the ideal properties of a carrier for clinical use [97]. Phagocytosis and accumulation of polyacrylamide spheres in large secondary lysosomes induced reversible necrotic cellular alterations in liver, together with changes in liver and spleen weights and enhanced autophagocytosis of macrophages [98-100]. In dogs, complete hepatic artery embolisation of the liver with non-degradable microparticulate polyvinyl alcohol foam particles (0.25 to 1 mm in diameter) has been shown to result in both deterioration of hepatic function for 4 weeks and focal infarctions [101]. Proximal dearterialisation combined with distal embolisation using 50 micron-sized non-degradable polystyrene particles induced liver infarction in pigs [102]. Surgical dearterilisation of the liver for the treatment of hepatic malignancies has been shown to be of limited value, because of the rapid opening of preexisting collaterals. For more information, see the review by Ackerman [5], who considers various therapeutic techniques related to tumour blood supply, including hepatic artery ligation and dearterialisation.

Manufacture and Properties of Colloidal Drug Carriers

Methods for the preparation of monodispersed polymer particles, with or without drugs, have been reviewed in the monographs edited by Widder and Green [95], Illum and Davis [103] and Davis et al. [104]. In this chapter, only a number of microsphere products will be considered for review, which have been selected based upon their clinical potential. For an extensive overview of the incorporation of more than 70 drugs into biodegradable colloidal carriers the reader is referred to Tomlinson [78,103].

Albumin Microspheres

In our laboratory, albumin microspheres of various sizes and composition are usually prepared by producing a water-in-oil emulsion followed by protein chain cross-linking with the use of heat [48-52,90,105-109] or chemical agents [41,45,47,78,110,111-114]. A disadvantage of cross-linking by thermal denaturation is due to the thermo-instability of some drugs; e.g., doxorubicin decomposes at 135° C [95,106]. On the other hand, methotrexate is inactivated using 2,3-butadione as cross-linking agent [43]. In the oil phase, the hydrophobic regions of albumin will be exposed externally to the surface, thus creating hydrophobic surface characteristics after fixation [40,47,104]. Dispersing an aqueous albumin-drug suspension in polymethylmethacrylate or polyoxyethylene-polyoxypropylene solutions yielded more hydrophilic microspheres [110].

In general, high payloads are observed for the incorporation of highly water-soluble compounds into albumin spheres. The methods, however, are unsuitable for the incorporation of a large amount of poorly water-soluble drug into a minimum of microspheres since, firstly, the entrapping capacity is restricted to the solubility of the drug in the presence of albumin and their oil/water partition coefficients, and secondly, small aqueous volumes are usually used. Microsuspension-emulsion techniques have therefore been developed in our laboratory, enabling the incorporation of cytostatic drugs as an undissolved crystalline compound in a reproducible manner [131]. Another important factor influencing the biodistribution of crosslinked albumin microspheres is the extent of swelling after hydration, which leads to an increase in sphere diameter of 20-80% depending upon particle size and payload of drug [47,113].

Biodegradation of heat or chemically stabilised albumin microspheres can be easily controlled by changing the degree of crosslinking [115]. Spheres produced with glutaraldehyde concentrations of 2% or more, for example, are no longer susceptible to *in vitro* (chymo)trypsin digestion [116,117]. McVie et al. [43] entrapped 0.4% glutaraldehyde stabilised albumin microspheres (15-35 microns in diameter) in lungs of mice which degraded after 6 to 7 days. Similar results were observed in rat livers. By contrast, albumin microspheres cross-linked with 1% glutaraldehyde were even found in mouse lungs 11 months after systemic injection [41,45].

Acute toxicity studies with albumin microspheres [115] illustrated that intravenous bolus injections of 37 micron microspheres of up to 40 mg/kg did not cause significant visible changes in mice (LD50 > 200 mg/kg [80]), rabbits and dogs (LD50 around 200 mg/kg [115]). Larger doses, however, induced laborious breathing and sometimes death due to pulmonary embolisation. To summarise, systemic toxic effects represent primarily the sequelae of embolic ischaemia rather than direct chemical toxicity induced by catabolisation by, e.g., mononuclear phagocytes. Apparently, the formation of aggregates in the bloodstream strongly influences the degree of acute toxicity after i.v. injection of microspheres [118]. Systemic delivery of microspheres (above 7 micron in diameter) intended not to pass through the target cicula-tion or to localise in the RES [49,81], resulted in a homogeneous saturation of the target tissue, but with ischaemia of the microvasculature [80]. Large albumin microspheres (15-35 microns) have been used for lung scans at dosages up to 50 mg per patient without reports of significant toxicity [115]. Entry of albumin microspheres (15-25 microns) to the rabbit liver by arterial access was acceptable with amounts up to 2 to 4 mg/kg, larger amounts or particles greater than 25 micron caused severe irreversible damage to the liver [43]. Following intra-arterial delivery, microspheres of approximately 25 micron (0.4% glutaraldehyde stabilised) could be administered in doses of 1.0 mg per patient without causing any foreign body toxicity [43].

Carbohydrate and Gelatin Microspheres

A reasonable alternative to poly(lactide) spheres are polycarbonate carriers, since they are claimed to be less toxic. Requirements for carbohydrate microspheres are identical to those for albumin spheres. A unique use of carbohydrate polymers for cancer chemotherapy has been described for intra-arterial coadministration of degradable starch microspheres (DSM or Spherex) as a transient blocking agent with cytostatic drugs [119]. There exist two major differences between carbohydrate/gelatin and albumin; firstly, the protein binding of drugs to gelatin is weaker, and secondly, carbohydrate/gelatin is gelled by cooling [120].

Starch microspheres ranging from 6 up to 90 microns in diameter form occlusive hydrophilic gels after intra-arterial delivery. Up to the present, most studies have used co-infusion of drugs together with large serum alpha-amylase biodegradable starch microspheres of approximately 40 micron in diameter. These spheres showed *in vivo* half-lives of 15 to 30 minutes for intra-arterial occlusion therapy of hypervascular tumours [121,122]. During *in vivo* degradation, Spherex microspheres maintain their size and shape until they finally collapse, due to a higher degree of cross-linkage at the periphery of the spheres [119]. It can be anticipated that starch will be non-immunogenic in the native soluble form, and all immunological tests performed

support this assumption [98].
The actual incorporation of drugs into the matrix of small as well as large starch microspheres has been poorly studied. Recently, magnetic microspheres of 1.0 micron have been prepared by entrapping magnetite microcrystals into dextran matrices [88]. Covalent coupling of monoclonal antibodies to the surface of these magnetic starch spheres makes them suitable for cell separation in a continuous flow system. Mitomycin C has been encapsulated successfully into gelatin/dextran microspheres of 0.28 and 15 micron in diameter [123]. *In vitro* and *in vivo* release of entrapped mitomycin C showed a half-life of about 30 hours. After intramuscular injection, small sized (0.28 micron in diameter) spheres accumulated in the regional lymph nodes, whereas following intravenous delivery these starch particles were found primarily in the liver. Intravenous infusion of 15 micron starch microspheres leads to an accumulation in the lungs for more than 24 hours as determined with ^{131}I-labelled microspheres [123].
Gelatin microspheres with a diameter between 0.1 and 0.8 micron are made using a desolvation and hardening technique [120], and were observed to be phagocytosed *in vitro* by EMT 6, WEHI-3 and SP-1 tumour cell lines [120]. Little information is available concerning the antigenicity of gelatin-based products and they need further study [120]. Up to the present time, clinical use of starch and gelatin microspheres has been limited due to the low payloads of cytostatic agents which can be entrapped in or bound to the surface of the spheres. Using the suspension/emulsion procedure for incorporation of crystalline drug into the matrix of starch spheres, higher payloads are expected [130].

Acryloylated Polysaccharide Microparticles

To obtain more stable biodegradable starch microspheres, Artursson et al. [99] introduced acrylic groups into polysaccharides to obtain a polymerisable derivative. So far, only poly(acryl)-starch nanoparticles (0.2-1.6 microns) have been prepared by radical polymerisation of acrylic starch (maltodextrin, hydroxyethyl starch, glycogen or dextran) in water-in-oil emulsions [98]. The properties of poly(acryl)-starch spheres can be manipulated by varying the concentration of the different compounds in the polymerisation mixture, as reflected in the D-T-C values [98], a nomenclature described in detail by Edman et al. [100]. Low molecular weight drugs, however, can only be entrapped in those spheres by immobilisation in the acryloylated polysaccharide polymeric network, but this must be done without influencing their *in vivo* release properties. Poly(acryl)-starch nanoparticles are non-immunogenic and do not induce immunogenicity to entrapped autologous proteins [98]. If the promise from the data obtained so far is realised, these acryloylated polycarbonate particles may offer a new system for targeting at least macromolecules to the RES [124].

Polyester Microspheres

Poly(lactic acid), poly(glycolic acid) and their copolymers are now referred to as the representatives of synthetic biodegradable polymers for clinical use. Poly(d,l-lactide) and lactide/glycolide copolymer microspheres in the range of smaller than 2 [62,64] up to 400 microns [60,61,63] can be prepared by a solvent evaporation process [64]. In using this procedure, truly spherical matrices are synthesised which are suitable for *in vivo* delivery [63]. After systemic delivery, distribution studies in mice [63,118] with ^{14}C-labelled microspheres demonstrated that particles of 1 to 15 microns in diameter were primarily lodged in lungs (62%) and liver (16%) with no signs of an inflammatory reaction.
There are also findings that microspheres prepared from polylactic acid provoke severe inflammatory responses when injected into rabbit knee joints [125]. Microspheres within the 1 to 5 micron range appeared as well-defined spherical transparent colloidal particles phagocytised by lung cells, whereas those entrapped in liver were found in tissues surrounding the capillaries [118]. Hence, the more rigid poly(lactide) microspheres exhibit proper characteristics to be used for third-order drug targeting. Poly(d,l- lactide) microspheres are well tolerated at doses up to 20 mg per mice; larger doses, however, cause death of animals due to respiratory problems.
The biodegradability of spheres manufactured with aliphatic polyesters depends upon (stereo)chemical compositions of the poly-

mers used. Poly(l-lactide) carriers are practically non-degradable, with an *in vivo* half-life of 6.6 months [126]. In contrast, poly(l-lactide/glycolide) (50% l-lactide composition) disintegrates very rapidly by hydrolysis with a half-life of around 0.22 months after implantation in rats [126]. The high enclosure of residual dichloromethane after manufacture of poly(d,l-lactide) spheres is another problem that needs to be eliminated [60,61]. Due to the relative biocompatibility of polylactic acid polymers, poly-b-hydroxybutyric acid (PHB) has now been examined for use in drug delivery systems for, e.g., aclarubicin [67,68]. PHB is a linear homopolymer of D(-)-b-hydroxybutyric acid, which is biosynthesised and stored in various strains of bacteria [127]. Polylactic acid microspheres (1-15 microns) have been produced by Benita et al. [63], who embedded solid lomustine (CCNU) between the macromolecular chains. Since CCNU is temperature, water and pH sensitive, the biological activity of encapsulated CCNU was investigated *in vitro*. Colony formation assays with AKR leukaemia suggest that microspherical formulated CCNU was protected against decomposition [118]. In addition, acute toxicity studies in mice with CCNU-loaded carriers concluded that entrapping of lomustine into a polylactide matrix significantly decreased systemic toxicity. Bissery et al. [128] evaluated the systemic therapeutic efficacy of polyester CCNU- loaded 3 micron spheres by life span increase in BD2F1 mice bearing Lewis Lung carcinomas. These studies showed that poly-b-hydroxybutyrate CCNU-loaded microspheres with a fast initial drug release (empty within 24 hours) had no effect, only slow CCNU releasing poly(d,l-lactide) microspheres (empty within 7 days) increased the survival of LL bearing mice over controls.

Ethylcellulose and Poly(d,l-lactide-co-glycolide) Microcapsules

Under certain conditions, ethylcellulose dissolved in an organic solvent accumulates over particles of water-soluble compounds to form a solid semipermeable capsular wall, a process known as coacervation or phase separation. Kato et al. [58,59] have developed an intra-arterial chemoembolisation system which utilised mitomycin C or cisplatin-loaded ethylcellulose microcapsules (200 micron in diameter), and they have reported encouraging clinical responses to such therapy. A disadvantage of this carrier, however, is the extremely stable envelope around the core. Madoulé et al. [129] described the appearance of foreign body reactions 8 days after loco-regional delivery, indicating little degradation *in vivo* over this period. The encapsulation of water-soluble drugs into poly(d,l- lactide) using the solvent evaporation process was therefore initiated [60,61]. The disadvantageous diffusion of cisplatin into the aqueous phase was prevented by saturation of the dispersing phase with the drug. Although an injectable drug-polymer system able to provide a fast and adjustable release could be produced, it is noted that saturating the aqueous phase with cisplatin leads to high losses of expensive cytostatics. It can be argued that the method of phase separation for the encapsulation of cisplatin and other water-soluble anticancer drugs into poly(d,l-lactide-co-glycolide) microcapsules could be a solution to create proper sustained release devices [130-132].

Drug-in-Oil Emulsions

Konno et al. [75,133-137] discovered that when the lipid contrast medium, Lipiodol, was administered arterially, it remained selectively in solid tumours. Based upon differences between the neovasculature of solid tumours and vasculature of normal tissues: e.g., lack of a lymphatic clearance system, absence in neovasculature of receptors to vasoconstrictors, and enhanced permeability to macromolecules and their prolonged retardation in extra-capillary spaces, it is concluded that oily anticancer drugs solubilised in Lipiodol can be utilised for solid tumour selective targeting [75,135]. Another advantage includes its enhanced visualisation on X-ray examinations, which also enables long-term follow-up.

It is known that intravenous injections of the high molecular weight anticancer agent copoly(styrene-maleic acid) conjugated to neocarzinostatin (SMANCS, Mr 17,000) induces marked antitumour effects in gastric and oesophageal cancer. In rabbits with hepatic VX-2 carcinoma, SMANCS dissolved in Lipiodol and administered via the hepatic artery [133], distributed throughout the entire normal arterial lumina with a gradual disappearance after 24 hours. Bioactive Lipiodol, however, was retained in tumour tissue and vessels for at least 7 days, whereas it was undetectable in any other organ. The use of ^{14}C-labelled derivatised Lipiodol [153] revealed remarkably high targeting ratios after injection; at 15 min 1000 times more and at 3 days 100 times more Lipiodol accumulated in tumour tissue compared to levels in most other organs or plasma. Its major excretion route appeared to be through bile and faeces. It is suggested that the non-tumorous liver adjacent to the VX-2 tumour contained relatively high levels of SMANCS as a result of continuous drug release from the drug-in-oil emulsion [133,137]. Histologically, massive tumour necrosis and infiltration of inflammatory cells were found, and the survival time of treated animals was significantly increased, even though only a single-dose schedule was given for this highly malignant tumour [133]. At laparotomy, however, no significant differences in tumour size were observed between the groups.

In 1987, Konno and Maeda [136] extended this technique to other lipids. At 24 hours the greatest retention in tumour tissues was observed with a semisynthetic medium-chain triglyceride/SMANCS emulsion (between 4.9 and37% of injected dose). No deleterious side-effects were observed on critical organs (Lipiodol: LD50 = 1.6 ml/kg dog i.v.; SMANCS: LD50 = 3.4 mg/kg mouse i.v.). Moreover, with angiotensin II, a larger volume of oily SMANCS-Lipiodol emulsion could be delivered to the tumour [75]. Taniguchi et al. [137] suspended doxorubicin, 5-fluorouracil and mitomycin C into Lipiodol, and observed that *in vitro* 40% of 5-FU was released from the drug-in-oil emulsion within 24 hours, whereas the release of doxorubicin and mitomycin C was much slower. It was suggested that, firstly, the release rate of anticancer drugs can be controlled by modifying the drug dosage and formulation and, secondly, Lipiodol can be used as a vehicle in combined drug cancer therapy [137]. In conclusion, the treatment of solid tumours, in particular, primary and metastatic liver cancer, using hydrophobic-polymer conjugated macromolecular anticancer drugs (SMANCS) suspended in oil (Lipiodol), may be a new direction for the development of tumour-selective chemotherapy [77,135].

Release and Diffusion Characteristics of Drugs from Colloidal Carriers

There have been an increasing number of studies attempting to develop drug delivery systems in which the drug can be utilised most effectively and safely by optimising the drug incorporation and release rates. Drug release from different devices takes place via a very complicated process, and although extensively studied, it is still unclear in many details. Factors that determine the release rate are: surface erosion, total particle digestion, drug diffusion and desorption, device geometry, drug load and leaching [98]. Another most important parameter in release behaviour is the water uptake of the polymeric network. In this chapter only a very short overview can be given on this subject. Excellent reviews on drug release which highlight the major features have been written by Chien [138], Roorda et al. [139] and Hadgraft and Guy [140].

Matrix Devices

Most microspheres consist of a monolith of polymer in which an amount of drug is dispersed throughout the network or matrix. If the polymeric network is in equilibrium swelling, there is only an efflux of drug, and transport occurs from the surface towards the centre according to the normal Fickian laws of diffusion. Thus, an inward moving boundary of dissolution recedes into the sphere that creates a drug concentration gradient [139,141]. Studies on drug release of doxorubicin from albumin microspheres [105-107] and of cisplatin from poly(d,l-lactide)-co-glycolide microspheres [60,61], respectively, showed that the Higuchi equations [141] provided a reasonable fit to the experimental data for the initial as well as terminal release phases. Albumin microspheres [45,78,142], however, swell uncontrollably under non-equilibrium situations, resulting in non-Fickian release behaviour. At the onset of drug release, the rate of delivery is very high for a short period, e.g., 80-95% of built-in cisplatin, the so-called burst effect. Burst effects may also be a consequence of a very high drug content in the periphery of the sphere [63,78,142]. McVie et al. [43] have described the biphasic release patterns of 5-FU, methotrexate and cisplatin-loaded human albumin spheres [78,142]. Mono-phasic first-order models were used to successfully fit the drug release profiles of CCNU-loaded poly(d,l-lactide) microspheres [63] and gelatin microcapsules carrying dextran-conjugates of mitomycin C [143].

Dissolution-Controlled Devices

In a dispersed matrix system, the rate of dissolution of the suspended drug particles may be so slow that dissolution becomes the rate-limiting step in the release process. Using this phenomenon, we entrapped dichlorobis-(aminomethyl)cyclohexane platina(II) (TNO-1, NSC 269608; solubility: 0.09 mg/ml saline), a cisplatin analogue with promising antitumour effects into albumin microshperes. Almost zero-order kinetics were achieved for the slow release phase and the burst effect was reduced by a factor 6.5 compared to cisplatin-loaded albumin spheres [142]. Biodegradable TNO-1-loaded albumin microspheres (10-25 microns in diameter) were administered through hepatic arterial catheters in rats with colonic carcinoma CC531 metastases (< 2mm) [144]. The anticancer effect was evaluated 2 weeks after injection. A significantly higher drug concentration within tumour nodules was achieved during angio-occlusion, while systemic peak plasma levels were reduced by 70-80% compared with systemic delivery. Histologically, massive tumour necrosis and infiltration of inflammatory cells were only observed in those rats treated with hepatic arterial chemotherapy (Fig. 4). This drug/microsphere combination is now available for preclinical evaluation.

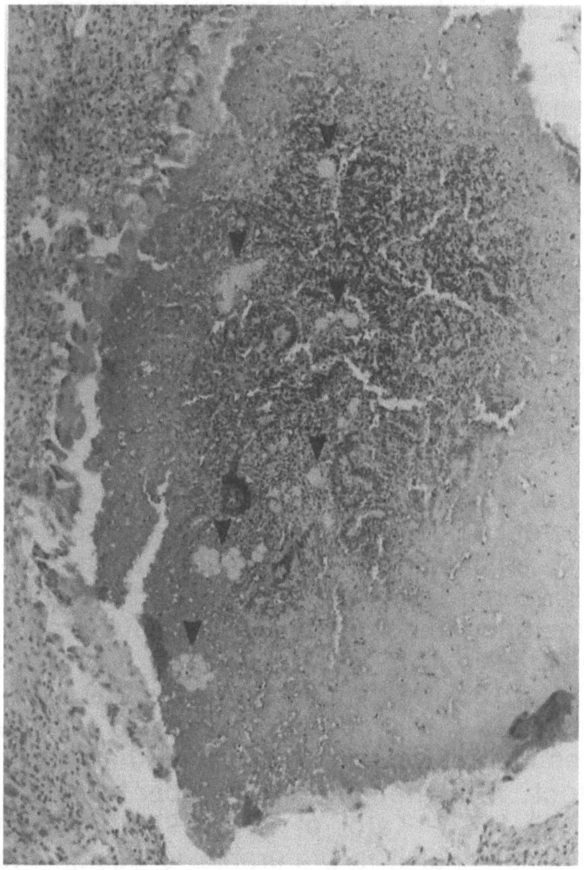

Fig. 4. Liver section with CC531 colonic carcinoma metastasis embedded in parafin and stained with hematoxylin and eosin 2 weeks after hepatic arterial injection of 4.0 mg albumin microspheres delivering a dose of 6.0 mg TNO-1 (NSC 269608)/kg of rat. Arrows show retained spheres surrounded by tumour necrosis and infiltration of inflammatory cells (x 100)

Capsular Devices

In aqueous media, water-soluble polymers, e.g., starch, dextrans, polyesters, formulated as capsular devices form a viscous gel-barrier on the surface of the sphere. Starch microspheres produced by emulsion polymerisation of soluble starch hydrolysate [119] swell in water and exhibit typical hydrogel characteristics [139]. During re-hydration, the central core is surrounded by some kind of rate limiting barrier, and a constant activity core may produce a constant concentration gradient over the barrier with zero-order release kinetics. Since the encapsulation of drugs into starch microspheres has been poorly studied, it cannot as yet be experimentally verified whether these conditions are fulfilled.

Devices with Non-Uniform Drug Distribution

Gupta et al. [105-107] created a sigmoidal concentration profile towards the centre of doxorubicin-loaded microspheres, probably caused by repeated washings. In this case, the non-uniform drug distribution through albumin networks showed an almost zero-order release of the drug.

Devices Controlled by Polymer Crystallinity

Poly-b-butyric acid (PHB) microspheres containing aclarubicin show nearly linear (zero-order) release profiles of the drug *in vitro* [67,68]. The high degree of crystallinity of poly-b-butyric acid is thought to explain the time-independent release [139]. The slow release rates of aclarubicin from PHB and polylactide microspheres could be enhanced over a wide range by incorporation of additives such as fatty acid esters [65,68], leading to channel formation and release profiles according to Higuchi equations [141].

In our opinion, the infusion of drug-loaded spheres [41,45,47,78,110-116] is the most reliable technique for loco-regional chemoembolisation if compared with the co-infusion of cytostatic drugs either with empty starch spheres [53-57,145] or Lipiodol [40,133,135,136,146]. On the other hand, extremely low or short high dose rapid release rates did not improve the desired therapeutic effect in selective anticancer therapy [65,68,128]. Kato et al. [59] therefore proposed that it is preferable to design the release of the encased drugs at a prolonged high dose rapid rate after devices reach the target by embolisation. The *in vivo* experiments of Bissery et al. [128], however, contradicted these suggestions, they demonstrated that CCNU-loaded poly (d,l-lactide) microspheres, releasing their drug content over 7 days, increased the survival of LL bearing mice over controls.

Clinical Potential of Chemoembolisation in Hepatic Cancer Chemotherapy

Non-Biodegradable Microcapsules: A Transcatheter Persistent Microparticulate Occlusive Technique

One of the first vehicles used for chemoembolisation were (non)biodegradable microcapsules prepared from ethylcellulose (225 micron in diameter) [58,59], and serum albumin (200-600 micron in diameter) [147], intended partly to induce infarction and partly cytotoxicity in tumours. The clinical experience of intravascular chemoembolisation with mitomycin C microcapsules, as a pre-operative or palliative measure, has been updated by Kato et al. [147]. Non-randomised trials, including 357 patients suffering from various advanced cancers who received one or two infusions of 29 mg (range 10-110 mg) encapsulated mitomycin C, have achieved a tumour response rate of 17% for hepatocellular carcinoma, 32% for renal cell carcinoma, and 69% for bladder tumours. As compared with mitomycin C, single infusions of built-in mitomycin C showed no significant difference in side effects; however, severe skin ulceration was seen in 9% of cases due to drug infusion into the hypogastric arteries. Comparative analysis according to treatment order, indicated a superiority of mitomycin C microcapsules combined with Gelfoam hepatic arterial embolisation over encapsulated mitomycin C alone, in terms of one-year survival rate (51.2% vs 16.9%) [147]. Although a significant palliation can be achieved with this aggressive modality, its value as a pre-operative measure to make organ-preserving surgery possible remains uncertain due to both the induction of extensive liver infarcts and inability of repeated dosing [101,102].

Biodegradable Rigid Microspheres: A Transcatheter Semi-Transient Microparticulate Occlusive Technique

There are only a limited number of clinical studies concerning HAI of drug-loaded microspheres within the 10 to 25 micron range. Preclinical evidence suggests, however, that it is appropriate to continue the use of these devices for chemoembolisation [148]. Since standard hepatic artery anatomy is present in only 50-60% of cases, radionuclide angiography with Tc-99m macroaggregated or microspherical albumin provides the necessary information for correct positioning of hepatic artery catheters [149] Hepatic artery radionuclide flow studies and hepatic angiography have shown that hepatic metastases tend to be hypervascular relative to surrounding hepatic parenchyma, and tumours in the 8.0 cm range possess a hypovascular core and hypervascular rim [43,150,151]. The finding of 25-40% of patients showing neoplastic lesions with no increased uptake, or else a high degree of arterio-venous shunting [152], and extra-hepatic abdominal flow [153-154], underlines the prerequisite for patient screening and selection for therapy [43]. Willmott and Cummings [117,155] injected doxorubicin-loaded albumin microspheres directly into solid Sp107 breast carcinoma growing subcutaneously in rats. They observed an increase of its antitumour effect compared with the same amounts of doxorubicin given intratumourally in solution [155]. Intra-arterial renal delivery of doxorubicin-loaded microspheres (20-40 microns in diameter [117]) in rabbits resulted in an uptake of 95% of injected spheres within the first renal capillary bed encountered [156], together with elevated renal tissue levels of doxorubicin [94], and 9 times lower peak plasma levels as compared with systemic free drug delivery [157]. In addition, intra-arterial chemoembolisation using mitomycin C-loaded albumin microspheres (45 micron in diameter) in rabbits bearing VX-2 hepatic lesions showed a remarkable tumour regression, if compared with free drug systemic delivery [157]. In humans, mitomycin C-loaded albumin microspheres given intraarterially for inoperable hepatic colorectal cancer with particular reference to a comparison with continuous infusion of mitomycin C and 5-FU, had superiority in response rate (68.4% vs 46.2%) and survival rate (15.6 $\pm$ 7.6 vs 8.6 $\pm$ 3.2 months); however, no effects on longevity were seen in patients with metastases from gastric and gallbladder primary tumours [158,159].

Central portions of solid tumours are usually relatively hypovascular and probably contain hypoxic cells [160]. Hypoxic cells are resistant to radiation, whereas the hypoxic state is particularly susceptible to some drugs which are activated by bioreduction, including mitomycin C. Besides the development of chronic hypoxia, acute hypoxia can be induced in solid hepatic tumours through transient or persistent occlusion of the capillary bed using microspheres. Mitomycin C shows 5 to 10-fold greater cell killing in hypoxic versus oxic cells [161]. Thus, transcatheter embolisation of the arteriolar capillary bed with mitomycin C-loaded albumin microspheres may improve the antitumour effect. Moreover, in the treatment of hepatic tumours by hyperthermia the effectiveness of heating at the capillary level could be improved by arterial chemoembilisation using starch microspheres Our studies have been focused on the use of cispatin-loaded albumin microspheres (15-25 micron diameter), containing 47-52% loading by weight of cisplatin. Preliminary phase I clinical trials have been conducted with the aim to examine the pharmacokinetics and pharmacodynamic advantages of administration of cisplatin built-in microspheres during hepatic artery infusion [45]. Nine pharmacokinetic studies were performed in 2 patients with advanced hypervascular hepatic metastases, which entered a 4-weekly dose-escalating study receiving 3 to 6 courses of cisplatin-loaded microspheres with dosages ranging from 10 up to 100 mg CDDP/m^2. Satisfactory arterial position of the catheter into tumour beds was confirmed by noting distribution patterns of 99mTc-labelled albumin spheres after injection. Typical pharmacokinetic curves after intra-arterial controlled delivery of cisplatin-loaded microspheres are included in Figure 5. They show that the curves of free and total platinum did not diverge rapidly reflecting a sustained delivery of the drug. Total platinum levels increased rapidly after infusion due to burst effects, followed by a normal biexponential decay curve, which did not vary from those obtained after conventional unformulated cisplatin given systemically or by HAI [163,164]. However, pharmacokinetic parameters of ultrafilterable platinum in plasma after HAI of cisplatin-loaded albumin microspheres at 100 mg/m^2 were significantly different from free drug levels after systemic or HAI delivery at the same dosages [163,164]. In plasma free platinum could be still detected up to 5 days after matrix-associated drug delivery ($t1/2\beta$= 44.7 - 239.5 h) and the shape of the prolonged β-phase suggested a sustained influx of cisplatin into the plasma compartment. Toxicities were therefore minimal, and the cumulative urinary excretion of platinum after 48 hours was about 30% of the dose.

Biodegradable Soft Microspheres: A Transcatheter Transient Occlusive Technique

A different chemoembolisation approach is the co-infusion of degradable starch microspheres (DSM, 40-45 microns in diameter) and drugs, e.g., mitomycin C, via the hepatic

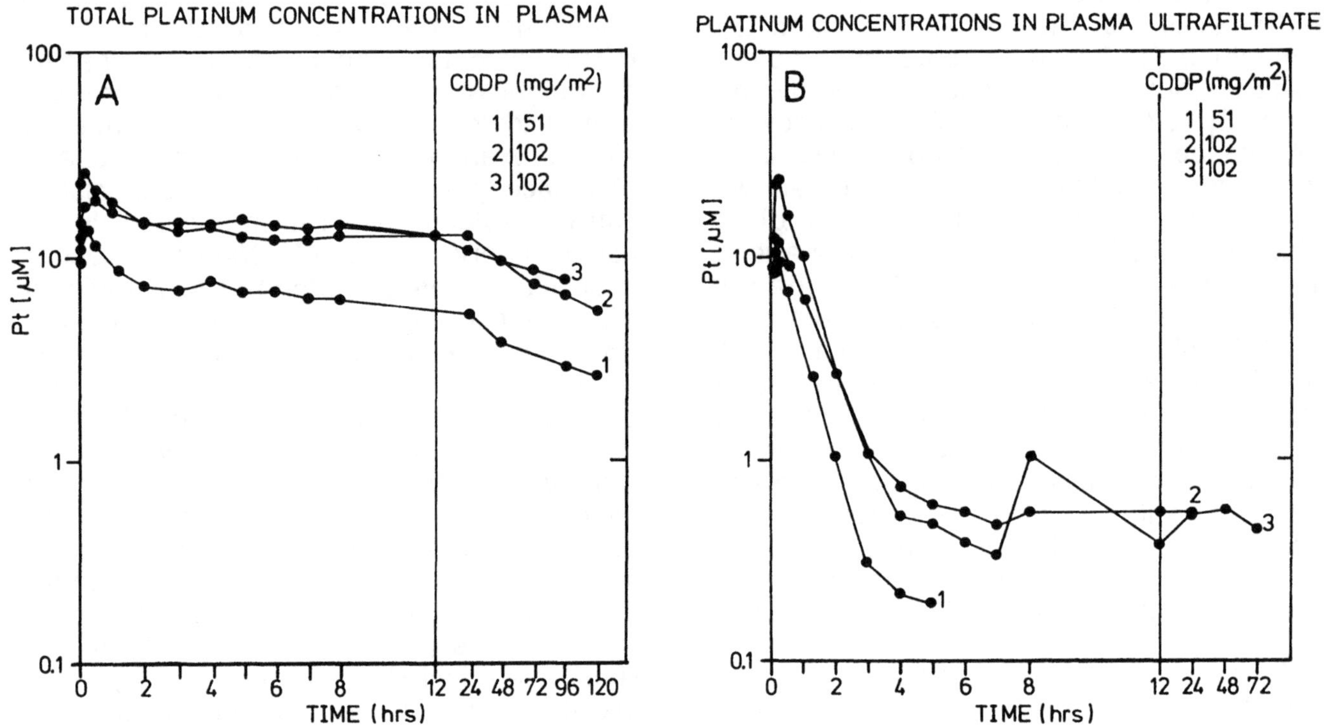

Fig. 5. Semilogarithmic plots of total platinum (A) and ultrafilterable platinum (B) versus time in a patient with sarcoma metastatic to liver, given cisplatin-loaded microspheres (10-25 μm; 47-52% loading by weight of CDDP; 0.4% glutaraldehyde stabilised) by intra-arterial hepatic infusions

artery, which produces acceptable systemic toxicity with maximal hepatic drug uptake [190]. Intra-arterial infusion of DSM temporarily obstructs the blood flow at the precapillary arterioles for 15-30 min, and is related to: 1) the density of the arteriolar capillary networks; 2) the number of starch spheres injected [54,122,165]; 3) arterial-blood flow, and 4) dose-dependent arterio-venous shunting events [121,153]. The relationship between flow reduction and amount of DSM administered, however, is non-linear [121,122], and appropriate doses of DSM for each treatment have to be individualised both to the patient's symptoms and computer-generated flow indices [193]. For this purpose, Starkhammer et al. [153] developed a reliable method for continuous monitoring of arterio-venous shunting after DSM infusion or collateral flow control.

The therapeutic efficacy of transient repeatable intratumoural ischaemia, in terms of response rate and survival, has been studied in a variety of drug-starch microsphere co-infusions. The pharmacokinetic advantage for this approach has been conclusively proven in phase I-II studies on previously treated patients. In all cases it has been demonstrated that systemic exposure can be decreased for each of the following drugs: 30-90% for BCNU [54,122], 21-42% for doxorubicin [145], 34% for FUDR [167], 15-60% for mitomycin C [121,167,168], due to greater hepatic drug retention. Moreover, arterial co-infusion of DSM increased the hepatic extraction of mitomycin C from 5-10% (HAI) to 40-45% after chemoembolisation [121]. In uncontrolled preliminary clinical studies most patients with malignant hepatic tumours (30-58%) have responded to intra-arterial embolisation using starch microspheres with either mitomycin C or doxorubicin [153,158,166,169-171]. In a multicentre Japanese phase II trial [172], entering 39 evaluable patients with primary liver cancers, hepatic arterial co-infusion of DSM and doxorubicin showed 2 complete responses (CR), 14 partial responses (PR), 22 minimal responses (MR) and 1 progressive disease (PD), giving an overall response rate of 41%. Transient occlusion of mitomycin C with DSM in 46 evaluable patients with secundary liver cancers resulted in 1 CR, 26 PR, 16 MR, and 16 stable diseases (SD), giving an overall response rate of 48.7%. The proof of its effectiveness, in terms of long-term superiority of DSM chemoembolisation over HAI therapy, is currently being studied in the scope of a prospective and randomised phase III trial with control groups [172]. So far, transient occlusion with DSM improved the therapeutic index, but the increase in tumour response seems to be insufficient to produce permanent tumour regression or prolonged survival [167,168]. The overall therapeutic benefit of repeated DSM chemotherapy administered via HAI, is a convenient palliation for metastatic or hepatocellular liver disease with some improvement in short-term control.

Transient Chemoembolisation with Concomitant Use of Vasoconstrictors

Newly formed blood vessels in neoplasms tend to be deficient in medial smooth muscle, contain a primitive fenestrated endothelial lining [173,174], and appear in many instances to be less responsive to systemically administered vasoactive drugs, e.g., adrenaline [175], noradrenaline [176]. For a review the reader is referred to Ackerman [5]. On the other hand, calcium antagonists, e.g., verapamil or nifedipine, induce an increased tumour blood flow regardless of the sites of the lesions [177]. Recent investigations have shown that angiotensin II possesses the ability to dramatically alter the distribution of blood in liver to further favour metastatic lesions [178]. Effects of angiotensin II co-infused with 5-FU and empty albumin spheres (20-40 microns in diameter) on systemic exposure of 5-FU have been studied in 9 patients with advanced colorectal hepatic cancer. Despite significant systolic blood pressure increase, no reduction in systemic exposure of 5-FU could be obtained compared with pharmacokinetic parameters after systemic infusion at the same dose level [93]. Although a negligible base line shunting was observed studying 5 other patients [179], in our opinion, the loss of regional advantage may be due to both a semi-transient occlusion of the 5-FU load within the microvasculature, and saturation of the hepatic extraction of 5-FU [180,181].

Drug-in-Oil Emulsions: A Transcatheter Oily Embolisation Technique

In non-randomised trials various solid human tumours, including metastatic liver cancer and cancers of lung, gallbladder and pancreas, have been treated by loco-regional therapy with drug-in-Lipiodol emulsions [77]. SMANCS, aclarubicin and mitomycin C in Lipiodol as single agent therapy or in mixtures were administered by catheterising the celiac or hepatic artery under X-ray monitoring in 216 patients with hepatocellular carcinoma. Konno and others [74,133,135] reported remarkable antitumour effects using this targeting schedule, serum AFP and tumour size both decreased in 91% of cases. No major side effects, such as bone marrow suppression or liver toxicity, were observed due to selective drug targeting to the tumour [133]. Ohtsuka et al. [76] noted that SMANCS/Lipiodol could be delivered to the metastatic lesions of the lymph nodes via the gastric artery, but not via lymphatic routes. Nakamura et al. [146] used doxorubicin-in-Lipiodol for transcatheter oily chemoembolisation. Cumulative survival rates for 100 patients with unresectable hepatoma were 53.8% for 1 year and 36.5% for 2 years, while 104 patients undergoing HAI without Lipiodol had 1 and 2-year survival rates of 45.2% and 16.3%, respectively. The lack of controlled trials (phase I-II), however, makes clinical assessment of transcatheter oily chemoembolisation impossible at the present time. The published studies generally indicate that the treatments were well tolerated, and produced some limited success in terms of tumour response.

Conclusions

Non-surgical treatments must still be considered palliative and rarely, if ever, curative. It is therefore essential to evaluate in an objective manner the effect on quality of life of any of these transcatheter occlusive techniques. If resection is not feasible, the vascularity of the tumour and anatomy of the hepatic artery should be assessed by angiography. Any patient demonstrating a definite flow of Tc-99m

macroaggregated albumin to the lungs or gastrointestinal tract should be excluded from therapy. Careful, elaborate and objective randomised comparisons of techniques should be executed before the optimal matrix-associated drug schedule can be recommended for inclusion in future treatment strategies.
It is unlikely that arterial delivery of drug-loaded colloidal carriers will ever constitute a solitary hepatic tumour therapy, but it may be of use in controlling regional metastasis to make organ-preserving surgery possible.

Acknowledgements

We are grateful to Dr. C. Hoefnagels for providing liver scans, to Dr. A.C. Begg for helpful suggestions and discussions. We gratefully acknowledge the support of the Netherlands Cancer Foundation KWF (grant No. NKI 86-6).

REFERENCES

1 Whitely HW Jr: Advanced colon and rectum cancer. In: Stearns M (ed) Neoplasms of the Colon, Rectum and Anus. Wiley, New York 1980 pp 101-113

2 Fortner JG, Silva JS, Cox EB et al: Multivariate analysis of a personal series of 247 patients with liver metastases from colorectal cancer. Ann Surg 1984 (199): 317-324

3 Russell AH, Peltom J, Regeis CE et al: Adenocarcinoma of the colon: an autopsy study with implications for new therapeutic strategies. Cancer 1985 (56): 1446-1451

4 Bragg DG: Angiography of hepatic neoplasms: a review. Int J Radiat Oncol Biol Phys 1976 (1): 965-971

5 Ackerman NB: The blood supply of liver metastases. In: Weiss L, Gilbert HA (eds) Liver Metastasis. G.K. Hall Med Publ Boston 1982 pp 96-125

6 Kemeny N: Role of chemotherapy in the treatment of colorectal carcinoma. Sem Surg Oncol 1987 (3): 190-214

7 Moertel CG: Chemotherapy of gastrointestinal cancer. N Engl J Med 1978 (229): 1049-1052

8 Labianca R, Pancera G, Beretta GD et al: Advanced colorectal cancer: polychemotherapy with cisplatin (CDDP) and 5FU vs 5FU alone. Results of a randomized study. Proc ECCO 1987 (4): A162

9 Windschill H, Scott M, Schutt A et al: Randomized phase II studies in advanced colorectal carcinoma: A North Central Cancer Treatment Group Study. Cancer Treat Rep 1983 (67): 1001-1008

10 Daly JM, Kemeny N. Therapy of colorectal hepatic metastases. Important Adv Oncol 1986: 251-268

11 Bedikian AY: Regional and systemic chemotherapy for advanced colorectal cancer. Dis Colon Rectum 1983 (26): 327-332

12 Lokich JJ, Bothe A, Zipoli T et al: Constant infusion schedule for adriamycin: A phase I-II clinical trial of a 30-day schedule by ambulatory pump delivery system. J Clin Oncol 1983 (1):24-28

13 Petrelli N, Herrora L, Stulc J et al: A phase III study of 5-fluorouracil (5-FU) versus 5-FU + methotrexate (MTX) versus 5-FU + high dose leucovorin (CF) in metastatic colorectal adenocarcinoma. Proc ASCO 1986 (5):78

14 Chlebowski RT, Paroly WI, Pugh RP et al: Adriamycin given as a weekly schedule without a loading dose: clinically effective with reduced incidence of cardiac toxicity. Cancer Treat Rep 1980 (64):47-51

15 Benjamin RS, Wiernik PH, Bachur WR: Adriamycin chemoterapy-efficacy, safety and pharmacologic basis of an intermittent single high dosage schedule. Cancer 1974 (33):19-27

16 Cooper KR, Hough WK: Prospective study of the pulmonary toxicity of continuous infused bleomycin. Cancer Treat Rep 1981 (65):419-425

17 Lokich JJ: Phase II study of cis-diamminedichloroplatinum (II) administered as a constant five-day infusion. Cancer Treat Rep 1980 (64):905-908

18 Eksborg S, Cedermark BJ, Strandler H-S Intrahepatic and intravenous administration of adriamycin-a comparative pharmacokinetic study in patients with malignant liver tumours. Med Oncol Tumor Pharmacother 1985 (2): 47-54

19 Stephens FO: Pharmacokinetics of intra-arterial chemotherapy Recent Results Cancer Res 1983 (86): 1-12

20 Campbell TN, Howell SB, Pfeifle CE et al: Clinical pharmacokinetics of intraarterial cisplatin in humans. J Clin Oncol 1983 (1): 755-762

21 Lokich JJ: Introduction to the concept and practice of infusion chemotherapy In: Lokich JJ (ed) Cancer Chemotherapy by Infusion. Precept Press Inc, Chicago 1987 pp 3-11

22 Chen H-SG, Gross JF: Intra-arterial infusion of anticancer drugs:theoretic aspects of drug delivery and review of responses. Cancer Treat Rep 1980 (64): 31-40

23 Ensminger WD, Gyves JW: Pharmacologic studies of hepatic intra-arterial chemotherapy. Dev Oncol 1985 (30): 237-245

24 Kemeny N, Daly J, Reichman B et al: Intrahepatic or systemic infusion of fluorodeoxyuridine in patients with liver metastases from colorectal carcinoma. A randomized trial. Ann Intern Med 1987 (107): 459-465

25 Hohn D, Stagg R, Friedman M et al: The NCOG randomized trial of intravenous (iv) vs hepatic arterial (IA) FUDR for colorectal cancer metastatic to the liver. Proc ASCO 1987 (6): A333.

26 Posner MP, Belliveau JF, Weitberg AB et al: Continuous infusion cisplatinum and bolus 5-fluorouracil in colorectal carcinoma. Cancer Treat Rep 1987 (71): 975-977

27 Lee Y-TN: Systemic and regional treatment of primary carcinoma of the liver. Cancer Treat Rev 1977 (4): 195-212

28 Patt YZ, Boddie AW, Charnsangavej C et al: Hepatic arterial infusion with floxuridine and cisplatin: overriding importance of antitumor effect versus degree of tumor burden as determinants of survival among patients with colorectal cancer. J Clin Oncol 1986 (4): 1356-1364

29 Patt YZ, Charnsangavej C, Boddie AW et al: Regional-arterial therapy embolization in the management of various stages of colon cancer. Dev Oncol 1985 (30): 341-355

30 Sigurdson ER, Ridge JA, Kemeny N et al: Tumor and liver drug uptake following hepatic artery and portal vein infusion. J Clin Oncol 1987 (5): 1836-1840

31 Stribley KV, Gray BN, Chmiel RL et al: Internal radiotherapy for metastases II: The blood supply to hepatic metastases. J Surg Res 1983 (34):25-32

32 Collins JM: Pharmacologic rationale for regional drug delivery. J Clin Oncol 1984 (2): 498-504

33 Ensminger WD, Gyves JW: Regional chemotherapy of neoplastic diseases. Pharmacol Ther 1983 (21): 277-293

34 Ensminger WD, Rosowski A, Raso V et al: A clinical-pharmacological evaluation of hepatic arterial infusions of 5-fluoro-2-deoxyuridine and 5-fluorouracil. Cancer Res 1978 (38): 3784-3792

35 Taylor I, Bennett R, Sheriff S: The blood supply of colorectal metastases. Br J Cancer 1979 (390): 749-756
36 Sasaki Y, Imaoka S, Hasegawa Y et al: Distribution of arterial blood flow in human hepatic cancer during chemotherapy-Examination by short-lived 81mKr. Surgery 1985 (97): 409-414
37 Dingemans KP: B16 metastasis in mouse liver and lung II. Morphology. Invasion Metastasis 1988 (8): 87-102
38 Jain RK: Determinants of tumour blood flow: a review. Cancer Res 1988 (48): 2641-2658
39 Blanchard RJ, Grotenhuis I, La Fave JW et al: Blood supply to hepatic V2 carcinoma implants as measured by radioactive microspheres. Proc Soc Exp Biol Med 1965 (118):465-468
40 Gyves JW, Zeissman HA, Ensminger WD et al: Definition of hepatic tumor microcirculation by single photon emission computerised tomography (SPECT). J Nucl Med 1984 (25): 972-977
41 Burger JJ, McVie JG: Microspheres for tumour targeting of cytostatic drugs. Pharm Weekbl Sci Ed 1985 (7): 27
42 McVie JG, Hoefnagel CA, Burger JJ: Tumortargeting of cytostatic compounds using intra-arterial biodegradable microspheres. Annual Report 1985. Netherlands Cancer Institute, Amsterdam 1985 pp 83-84
43 McVie JG, Burger JJ, Hoefnagel C, Tomlinson E: The use of microspheres in the treatment of liver metastases. In: Van de Velde CJH, Sugarbaker PH (eds) Liver Metastasis; Basic Aspects, Detection and Management. Martinus Nijhoff Publ Dordrecht 1984 pp 313-323
44 Civalleri D, Scopinaro G, Simoni G et al: Starch microspheres-induced arterial flow redistribution after occlusion of replaced hepatic arteries in patients with liver metastases. Cancer 1986 (58):2151-2156
45 Noteborn HPJM, Varossieau F, Blanken G et al: Clinical pharmacokinetics of cisplatin in intra-arterial hepatic carrier-mediated delivery in treatment of metastatic liver cancer. In: Heller J (ed) Proc 15th Int Symp Controlled Release Bioactive Materials, Basle 1988, pp 127-128
46 Merkel C, Cagol PP, Da Pian PP et al.: Blood flow of experimental liver metastases in rat as evaluated by the locally injected 133-Xenon washout. Res Exp Med 1985 (185): 207-215
47 Burger JJ, Tomlinson E, McVie JG: Microparticles intended for microvascular blockage. Drug incorporation and release. In: Buri P, Gumma A (eds) Drug Targeting. Elsevier Sci Publ Amsterdam 1985 pp 81-94
48 Burgess DJ, Davis SS, Tomlinson E: Potential use of albumin microspheres as a drug delivery system. I. Preparation and in vitro release of steroids. Int Pharm 1987 (39): 129-136
49 Widder KJ, Senyei AE: Magnetic microspheres: A vehicle for selective targeting of drugs. Pharm Ther 1983 (20): 377-395
50 Widder KJ, Flouret G, Senyei AE: Magnetic microspheres: Synthesis of a novel parenteral drug carrier. J Pharm Sci 1979 (68): 79-82
51 Sugibayashi K, Morimoto Y, Nadai T et al: Drug-carrier property of albumin microspheres in chemotherapy. II. Preparation and tissue distribution in mice of microsphere entrapped 5-fluorouracil. Chem-Pharm Bull 1979 (27): 204-209
52 Rettenmaier MA, Stutton JA, Berman ML et al: Treatment of a syngenic rat tumor with magnetically responsive albumin microspheres labeled with doxorubicin or protein A. Gynecol Oncol 1987 (27): 34-43
53 Aronsen KF, Hellekant C, Holmberg J et al: Controlled blocking of hepatic artery flow with enzymatically degradable microspheres combined with oncolytic drugs. Eur Surg Res 1979 (11): 99-106
54 Dakhil S, Ensminger WD, Cho K et al: Improved regional selectivity of hepatic arterial BCNU with degradable microspheres. Cancer 1982 (50):631-635
55 Lindell B, Aronson K-F, Nosslin A et al: Studies in pharmacokinetics and tolerance of substances temporarily retained in the liver by microspheres embolization. Ann Surg 1978 (187): 95-99
56 Tuma RF: The use of degradable starch microspheres for transient occlusion of blood flow and for drug targetingf to selected tissues. In: Davis SS, Illum L, McVie JG, Tomlinson E (eds) Microspheres and Drug Therapy. Elsevier Sci Publ Amsterdam 1984 pp 189-203
57 Tuma RF, Forsberg JO, Agerup B: Enhanced uptake of actinomycin D in the dog kidney by simultaneous injection of degradable starch microspheres into the renal artery. Cancer 1982 (50): 1-5
58 Kato T, Nemoto R: Microencapsulation of Mitomycin C for intra-arterial infusion chemotherapy. Proc Jpn Acad 1978 (54): 413-417
59 Kato T, Unno K, Goto A: Ethylcellulose microcapsules for selective drug delivery. Meth Enzymol 1985 (112): 139-150
60 Spendlehauer G, Vert M, Benoit JP et al: Biodegradable cisplatin microspheres prepared by the solvent evaparation method: morphology and release characteristics. J Control Rel 1988 (in press)
61 Spendlehauer G, Veillard M, Benoit JP: Formation and characterization of cisplatin loaded poly(d,l-lactide) microspheres for chemoembolization. J Pharm Sci 1986 (75): 750-755
62 Tabata Y, Ikada Y: Activation of macrofage in vitro to acquire antitumor activity by a muramyl dipeptide derivative encapsulated in microspheres composed of lactide copolymer. J Control Rel 1987 (6): 189-204
63 Benita S, Benoit JP, Puisieux C et al: Characterization of drug-loaded poly(dl-lactide) microspheres. J Pharm Sci 1984 (73): 1721-1724
64 Bodmeier R, McGinity JW: The preparation and evaluation of drug-containing poly(dl-lactide) microspheres formed by the solvent evaporation method. Pharm Res 1987 (4): 465-471
65 Juni K, Ogata J, Matsui N et al: Control of release rate of bleomycin from polylactic acid microspheres by additives. Chem Pharm Bull 1985 (33): 1609-1614

66 Juni K, Ogata J, Matsui N et al: Modification of the release rate of aclarubicin from polylactic acid microspheres by using additives. Chem Pharm Bull 1985 (33) 1734-1738

67 Juni K, Nakano M, Kubota M: Controlled release of aclarubicin, an anticancer antibiotic, from poly-b-hydroxybutyric acid microspheres. J Control Rel 1986 (4): 25-32

68 Kubota M, Nakano M, Juni K: Mechanism of enhancement of the release rate of aclarubicin from poly-b-hydroxybutyric acid microspheres by fatty acid esters. Chem Parm Bull 1988 (36): 333-337

69 Lenearts V, Couvreur P, Christiaens-Leyh D et al: Degradation of poly(isobutylcyanoacrylate) nanoparticles. Biomaterials 1984 (5): 65-68

70 Gipps EM, Arshady R, Kreuter J et al: Distribution of polyhexyl cyanoacrylate nanoparticles in nude mice bearing human osteosarcoma. J Pharm Sci 1986 (75): 256-258

71 Douglas SJ, Illum L, Davis SS: Poly(butyl 2-cyanoacrylate) nanoparticles with differing surface charges. J Control Rel 1986 (3):15-23

72 Illum L, Kahn MA, Mak E et al: Evaluation of carrier capacity and release characteristics for poly(butyl 2-cyanoacrylate) nanoparticles. Int J Pharm 1986 (30): 17-28

73 Douglas SJ, Davis SS, Illum L: Nanoparticles in drug delivery. Crit Rev Ther Drug Carrier Syst 1987 (3): 233-261

74 Konno T: Targeting chemotherapy of hepatocellular carcinoma by arterial administration of anticancer agents dissolved in lipiodol. Gan To Kagaku Ryoho 1987 (14): 373-380

75 Konno T, Ohtsuka N, Yamasaki K et al: Targeting of anticancer chemotherapy utilizing the characteristic nature of the neovasculature of solid tumors. Gan To Kagaku Ryoho 1986 (13): 1448-1455

76 Ohtsuka N, Konno T, Miyauchi Y et al: Anticancer effects of arterial administration of the anticancer agent SMANCS with lipiodol on metastatic lymph nodes. Cancer 1987 (59): 1560-1565

77 Konno T, Maeda H, Iwai S et al: Selective targeting of anti-cancer drug and simultaneous image enhancement in solid tumors by arterially administered lipid contrast medium. Cancer 1984 (54): 2367-2374

78 Tomlinson E Microsphere delivery systems for drug targeting and controlled release. Int J Pharm Tech Prod Mft 1983 (4): 49-57

79 Illum L, Davis SS: Passive and active targeting using coloidal drug carrier systems. In: Buri P, Gumma A (eds) Drug Targeting. Elsevier Sci Publ Amsterdam 1985 pp 65-80

80 Widder KJ, Senyei AE, Ranney DF: Magnetically responsive microspheres and other carriers for the biophysical targeting of antitumour agents. Adv Pharmacol Chemother 1979 (16): 213-271

81 Burger JJ, Tomlinson E, De Roo JE et al: Technetium-99m labeling of albumin microspheres intended for drug targeting. Meth Enzymol 1985 (112): 43-56

82 Illum L, Davis SS: Effect of the nonionic surfactant Poloxamer 338 on the fate and deposition of polystyrene microspheres following intravenous administration. J Pharm Sci 1983 (72): 1086-1089

83 Illum L, Davis SS: The organ uptake of intravenously administered colloidal particles can be altered using a non-ionic surfactant (Poloxamer 338). FEBS Lett 1984 (167): 79-82

84 Wilkins DJ, Meyer PA: Studies on the relationship between the electrophoretic properties of colloids and their blood clearance and organ distribution in the rat. Brit J Exp Path 1966 (47): 568-576

85 Morimoto Y, Sugibayashi K, Okumura M et al: Biomedical applications of magnetic fluids. I. Magnetic guidance of ferro-colloid entrapped albumin microspheres for site-specific drug delivery in vivo. J Pharm Dyn 1981 (4): 624-631

86 Artursson P, Laakso T, Edman P: Acrylic microspheres in vivo. IX. Blood elimination kinetics and organ distribution of microparticles with different surface characteristics. J Pharm Sci 1983 (72): 1415-1420

87 Salky NK, Di Luzio NR, Levin AG et al: Phagocytic activity of the reticuloendothelial system in neoplastic disease. J Lab Clin Med 1967 (70): 393

88 Schroeder U, Stahl A, Salford LG: In: Davis SS, Illum L, McVie JG, Tomlinson E (eds) Microspheres and Drug Therapy. Elsevier Sci Publ Amsterdam 1984 p 427

89 Ranney DF: Pulmonary targeting with ferromagnetised albumin microsphere. Science 1985 (227): 182-183

90 Kramer PA, Burnstein T: Phagocytosis of microspheres containing an anticancer agent by tumour cells in vitro. Life Sci 1976 (19): 515-520

91 Kramer PA: Albumin microspheres as vehicles for achieving specificity in drug deliveries. J Pharm Sci 1974 (63): 1646-1647

92 Grislain P, Couvreur P, Lenaerts V et al: Pharmacokinetics and distribution of a biodegradable drug-carrier. Intern J Pharmaceut 1983 (15): 335-34515): 335-345

93 Goldberg JA, Kerr DJ, Willmott N et al: Pharmacokinetcs and pharmacodynamics of loco-regional 5-Fluorouracil (5-FU) in advanced colorectal liver metastases Br J Cancer 1988 (57): 186-189

94 Willmott N: Chemoembolization in regional cancer chemotherapy: a rationale Cancer Treatm Rev 1987 (14): 143-156

95 Widder KJ, Green R (eds): Drug and Enzyme Targeting. Meth Enzymol. Academic Press Inc, Orlando 1985 (112)

96 Freeman AI, Mayhew E: Targeted drug delivery. Cancer 1986 (58):573-583

97 Burgener FA, Gothlin JH: Angiography, microangiographic and hemodynamic evaluation of artery embolization in the rabbit. Invest Radiol 1978 (13):306-312

98 Edman P, Artursson P, Laakso T et al: Poly(cryl)-starch microspheres as drug carrier systems. In: Illum L, Davis SS (eds) Polymers in Controlled Drug Delivery. Wright, Bristol 1987 pp 87-98

99 Artursson P, Edman P, Laakso T et al: Characterization of polyacryl starch microparticles as carriers for proteins and drugs. J Parm Sci 1984 (73): 1507-1513

100 Edman P, Ekman B and Sjoholm I: Immobilization of proteins in microspheres of biodegradable polyacryldextrans. J Pharm Sci 1980 (69): 838-842
101 Chuang VP, Tsai C-C, Soo C-S et al.: Experimental canine hepatic artery embolization with polyvinyl alcohol foam particles. Radiology 1982 (145): 21-25
102 Stridbeck H, Lorelius L-E, Pritle TE: Development of colloidal circulation following distal embolization of hepatic artery in pigs. Cardiovasc Intervent Radiol 1984 (7): 240-244
103 Illum L, Davis SS (eds): Polymers in controlled drug delivery. Wright, Bristol 1987
104 Davis SS, Illum L, McVie JG, Tomlinson E (eds): Microspheres and Drug Therapy. Elsevier Sci Publ, Amsterdam 1984
105 Gupta PK, Hung CT, Perrier DG: Albumin microspheres. I. Release characteristics of adriamycin. Int J Pharm 1986 (33): 137-146
106 Gupta PK, Hung CT, Perrier DG: Albumin microspheres. II. Effect of stabilization temperature on the release of adriamycin. Int J Pharm 1986 (33): 147-153
107 Gupta PK, Gallo JM, Hung CT et al: Influence of stabilization temperature on the entrapment of adriamycin in albumin microspheres. Drug Dev Ind Pharm 1987 (13): 1471-1482
108 Widder KJ, Senyei AE, Sears B: Experimental methods in cancer therapeutics. J Pharm Sci 1982 (71): 379-387
109 Senyei AE, Driscoll CF, Widder KJ: Biophysical drug targeting; Magnetically responsive albumin microspheres. Meth Enzymol 1985 (112): 56-67
110 Longo WE, Iwata H, Lindheimer TA et al: Preparation of hydrophilic albumin microspheres using polymeric dispersing agents. J Pharm Sci 1982 (71): 1323-1328
111 Yapel AF Albumine microspheres: Heat and chemical stabilization. Method Enzymol 1985 (112): 3-18
112 McArdle CS, Lewi H, Hansell D et al: Cytotoxic-loaded albuminmicrospheres: a novel approach to regional chemotherapy. Br J Surg 1988 (75): 132-134
113 Burger JJ, Tomlinson E, Mulder EMA et al: Albumin microsheres for intra-arterial tumour targeting. I. Pharmaceutical aspects. Int J Pharm 1985 (23): 333-334
114 Chen Y, Willmott N, Anderson J et al: Comparison of albumin and casein microspheres as a carrier for doxorubicin. J Pharm Pharmacol 1987 (39): 978-985
115 Rhodos BA, Zolle I, Buchman JW et al: Radioactive albumin microspheres. Radiology 1983 (92): 1453-1460
116 Lee TK, Sokolski JD, Royer GP: Serum albumin beads: An injectible, biodegradable system for the sustained release of drugs. Science 1981 (213): 233-235
117 Willmott N, Cummings J, Stuart JFB et al: Adriamycin loaded albumin microspheres: Preparation, in vivo distribution and release in the rat. Biopharmacol Drug Dispos 1985 (6): 91
118 Bissery M-C, Valeriote F, Thies C: In: Davis SS, Illum L, McVie JG, Tomlinson E (eds) Microspheres and Drug therapy. Elsevier Sci Publ, Amsterdam 1984 pp 217-229
119 Lindberg B, Lote K, Teder H: Biodegradable starch microspheres-A new medical tool. In: Davis SS, Illum L, McVie JG, Tomlinson E (eds) Microspheres in Drug Therapy. Elsevier Sci Publ Amsterdam 1984 pp 153-188
120 Oppenheim RC: Gelatin microspheres as drug carrier systems. In: Illum L, Davis SS (eds) Polymers in Controlled Drug Delivery. Wright, Bristol 1987 pp 73-86
121 Gyves JW: Selective therapy of hepatic cancers using microspheres. In: Rosenthal CJ, Rotman M (eds) Plenum Press New York 1986 pp 67-69
122 Ensminger WD: Degradable starch microspheres. Dev Oncol 1984 (26):219-226
123 Sezaki H, Hashida M, Muranashi S: In: Optimization of drug delivery Munksgaard Copenhagen 1982 pp 316
124 Artursson P, Sjoholm I: Effect of opsonins on the macrophage uptake of polyacrylstarch microparticles. Int J Pharm 1986 (32): 165-170
125 Ratcliffe JH, Hunneyball IM, Smith A et al: Preparation and evaluation of biodegradable polymeric systems for the intra-articular delivery of drugs. J Pharm Pharmacol 1984 (36): 431-436
126 Miller RA, Brady JM, Cutright DE: Degradation rates of oral resorbable implants (polyactates and polyglycolates): rate modification with changes in PLA/PGA copolymer ratios. J Biomed Mat Res 1977 (11): 711-719
127 Senior DJ, Dawes EA: Poly-b-hydroxybutyrate biosynthesis and the regulation of glucose metabolism in Azotobacter beijerinckii. Biochem J 1971 (125): 55-56
128 Bissery MC, Valeriote FA, Thies C: Therapeutic efficacy of CCNU-loaded microspheres prepared from poly(d,l)lactide (PLA) or poly-B-hydroxybutyrate (PHB) against Lewis lung (LL) carcinoma. Proc Annu Meet Am Assoc Cancer Res 1985 (26): 355
129 Madoulé P, Trampont P, Roche A: Chemoembolization: principles and perspectives. J Microencaps 1984 (1): 21-25
130 Sanders LM, McRae GI, Vitale KM et al: Controlled delivery of an LH-RH analogue from biodegradable injectable microspheres. J Control Rel 1985 (2): 187-195
131 Sanders LM, Kent JS, McRae GI et al: Controlled release of a luteinizing hormone-releasing hormone analogue from poly(d,l-lactide-co-glycolide) microspheres. J Pharm Sci 1984 (73): 1294-1297
132 Makino K, Arakawa M, Kondo T: Preparation and in vitro degradation properties of polylactide microcapsules. Chem Pharm Bull 1985 (33):1195-1201
133 Maeda H, Konno T, Iwai K et al: Tumor selective drug delivery with lipid contrast medium (SMANCS/LIPIODOL): sustained antitumor effect, enhanced diagnostic value and quantification of dosage regiman. Gan To Kagaku Ryoho 1984 (4): 814-826
134 Iwai K, Maeda H, Konno T: Use of oily contrast medium for selective drug targeting to tumor:

enhanced therapeutic effect and X-ray image. Cancer Res 1984 (44): 2115-2121
135 Maeda H, Konno T: Tumor-targeted chemotherapy with lipid contrast medium and macro molecular anticancer agents theoretical considerations and clinical outcome. Gan To Kagaku Ryoho 1985 (12):773-782
136 Iwai K, Maeda H, Konno T et al: Tumor targeting by arterial administration of lipids: rabbit model with VX2 carcinoma in the liver. Anticancer Res 1987 (7): 321-327
137 Taniguchi H, Yamaguchi T, Takahashi T: Basic study of anti-cancer agents suspended in Lipiodol. Gan To Kagaku Ryoho 1986 (13): 255-260
138 Chien YW: In: Novel drug delivery systems. Marcel Dekker, New York 1982 p 663
139 Roorda WE, Bodde HE, De Boer AG et al: Synthetic hydrogels as drug delivery systems. Pharm Weekbl Sci Ed 1986 (8): 165-188
140 Hadgraft J, Guy RH: Release and diffusion of drugs from polymers. In: Davis SS, Illum L (eds) Polymers in Controlled Drug Delivery. Wright, Bristol 1987 pp 99-116
141 Higuchi T: Rate of release of medicaments from ointment base containing drugs in suspension. J Pharm Sci 1961 (50): 874-875
142 McVie JG, Meinema HA, Blanken-Aarsen GJ et al: Formulation of poorly water-soluble cytostatic platinum compounds using biodegradable microspheres. VIII.7.3 Annual Report 1987. Netherlands Cancer Institute, Amsterdam 1988 p 98
143 Yoshioka T, Hashida M, Muranishi S et al: Specific delivery of mitomycin C to the liver, spleen and lung: nano- and microspherical carries of gelatin. Int J Pharm 1981 (8): 131-141
144 Boutkan H, Ruevekamp M, Ter Berg RGM et al: Determination of the liver tumor load in colonic carcinoma metastasising to the liver: an experimental study in the rat. Surg Res Comm 1988 (3): 319-325
145 Teder H, Nilsson B, Jonsson K et al. : Hepatic arterial administration of doxorubicin (adriamycin) with or without degradable starch microspheres: a pharmacokinetic study in man. In: Hansen H (ed) Anthracyclines and Cancer Therapy. Elsevier Medica, Amsterdam 1983 pp 166-174
146 Nakamura H, Hashimoto T, Taguchi T et al.: Chemoembolization. Gan To Kagaku Ryoho 1987 (14): 1656-1663
147 Okamoto Y, Konno A, Togawa K et al: Arterial chemoembolization with cisplatin microcapsules. Br J Cancer 1986 (53): 369-375
148 Morimoto Y, Fujimoto S: Albumin microspheres as drug carriers. Crit Rev Ther Drug Carrier Syst 1985 (2):19-63
149 Kato T, Kazunari S, Abe R et al: Clinical trial of intravascular targeted chemotherapy (chemoembolization) with mitomycin C microcapsules. In: Taguchi T, Andrysek O (eds) New Trends in Cancer Chemotherapy with Mitomycin C. Excerpta Medica Ltd Tokyo 1987 pp 158-170
150 McVie JG, Burger JJ, Hoefnagel C, Tomlinson E: The use of microspheres in the treatment of liver metastases. Rev Oncol 1984 (24): 313-323
151 Zeissman HA, Thrall JH, Yang PJ et al: Hepatic arterial scintigraphy with Tc-99m-MAA Radiology 1982 (152): 167-172
152 Charnsangajev C, Carrasco C, Wallace S et al: Hepatic arterial flow distribution with hepatic neoplasms: significance in infusion chemotherapy. Radiology 1987 (165): 71-73
153 Starkhammer H, Hakansson L, Morales O et al: Effect of microspheres in intra-arterial chemotherapy. A study of arterio-venous shunting and passage od a labelled marker. Med Oncol Tumor Pharmacother 1987 (4):87-96
154 Wells JJ, Nostrant TT, Wilson JA et al: Gastroduodenal ulcerations in patients receiving selective hepatic artery infusion chemotherapy. Am J Gastroenterol 1985 (80): 425-429
155 Willmott N, Cummings J: Increased anti-tumour effect of adriamycin-loaded albumin microspheres is associated with anaerobic bioreduction of drug in tumour tissue. Biochem Pharmacol 1987 (36): 521-526
156 Wilmott N, Kerr D, Lewi H et al: Tissue localization of adriamycin (ADR) using albumin microspheres. Proc BACR 27th AGM 1987 p 189
157 Lewi H, Willmott N, Kerr DJ et al: Adriamycin loaded albumin microspheres: a new method of delivering cytotoxic therapy. Br J Surg 1986 (73): 612
158 Endoh F: Intra-arterial chemoembolization with albumin microspheres including mitomycin C in inoperable hepatic cancer. Nippon Geka Gakkai Zasshi 1987 (88): 584-593
159 Fujimoto S, Miyazaki M, Endoh F et al: Biodegradable mitomycin C microspheres given intra-arterially for inoperable hepatic cancer with particular reference to a comparison with continuous infusion of mitomycin C and 5-fluorouracil. Cancer 1985 (56): 2404-2410
160 Workman P: Hypoxic cells and cancer therapy. Cancer Topics 1982 (4):22-23
161 Workman P: New trends in targeted cancer chemotherapy. In: Domellöf L (ed) Drug delivery in cancer treatment. European School of Oncology Monograph Series. Springer-Verlag Berlin-New York 1987 pp 77-99
162 Tanaka Y, Murata T, Yoshida M et al: Enhancement of anti-tumour effects by arterial embolization combined with hyperthermia in the treatment of hepatic tumors. Gan To Kagaku Ryoho 1987 (14): 396-403
163 Vermorken JB, Van der Vijgh WJF, Klein I et al: Pharmacokinetics of free and total platinum species after short-term infusion of cisplatin. Cancer Treat Reports 1984 (68): 505-513
164 Stewart DJ, Benjamin RS, Zimmerman et al: Clinical pharmacology of intraarterial cis-diamminedichloroplatinum (II). Cancer Res 1983 (43):917-920
165 Ensminger WD, Gyves JW, Stetson P et al: Phase I study of hepatic arterial degradable starch microspheres and mitomycin. Cancer Res 1985 (45): 4464-4467

166 Pfeifle CE, Howell SB, Ashburn WL et al: Pharmacologic studies of intra-hepatic chemotherapy with degradable starch microspheres. Cancer Drug Deliv 1986 (3): 1-14
167 Ensminger WD: Degradable starch microspheres. Dev Oncol 1984 (26):219-226
168 Wollner IS, Walker-Andrews SC, Smith JE et al: Phase II study of hepatic arterial degradable starch microspheres and mitomycin. Cancer Drug Deliv 1986 (3): 279-284
169 Koike S, Fujimoto S, Endoh F et al: Combination intra-arterial chemotherapy with degradable starch microspheres and mitomycin C against inoperable hepatic metastases. Gan To Kagaku Ryoho 1988 (15):431-435
170 Itani K, Yoshikawa T, Tainaka K et al: Chemoembolization with degradable starch microspheres in malignant hepatic tumors. Gan To Kagaku Ryoho 1987 (14):388-395
171 Parker G, Regelson W: Biodegradable starch microspheres. In: Rosenthal CJ, Rotman M (eds) Clinical applications of continuous infusion chemotherapy and concomitant radiation therapy. Plenum Press, New York 1986 pp 51-66
172 Taguchi T: Clinical results of chemotherapy combined with degradable starch microspheres in a cooperative study. DSM study group in Japan (personal communication)
173 Wickersman JK, Barrett WP, Furakawa SB et al: An evaluation of the response of the microvasculature in tumours in C3H mice to vasoactive drugs. Bibl Anat 1977 (15): 291
174 Hammersen F, Endrich B, Messmer K: The fine structure of tumour blood vessels.I. Participation of non-endothelial cells in tumour angiogenesis. Int J Microcirc Clin Exp 1985 (4): 31-43
175 Burton MA, Gray BN: Distribution of blood flow in experimental hepatic tumours with noradrenaline and propranolol. Br J Cancer 1987 (56): 585-588
176 Iwaki A, Nagasue N, Kobayashi M et al: Intra-arterial chemotherapy with concomittant use of vasoconstrictors for liver cancer. Cancer Treat Rep 1978 (62): 145-146
177 Kaelin WG, Shrivastav S, Shand DG et al: Effect of verapamil on malignant tissue blood flow in SMT-2A tumor-bearing rats. Cancer Res 1982 (42): 3944-3949
178 Sasaki Y, Imaoka S, Hasegawa Y et al: Changes in distribution of hepatic blood flow by intraarterial infusion of angiotensin II in human hepatic cancer. Cancer 1985 (55): 311-316
179 Goldberg JA, Bradnam MS, Kerr DJ et al: Arterio-venous shunting of microspheres in patients with colorectal liver metastases: errors in assessment due to free pertechnetate and the effect of angiotensin II. Nucl Med Comm 1988 (in press)
180 Boublil JL, Milano G, Khater R et al: Continuous 5-day regional chemotherapy by 5-fluorouracil in colon carcinoma: pharmacokinetic evaluation. Br J Cancer 1985 (52):15-20
181 Milano G, Boublil JL, Khater R et al: 5-FU pharmacokinetics during locoregional treatment in patients with colorectal carcinoma. EORTC Symposium on Continuous Infusion Chemotherapy, March 1, 1985. Brussels 1985: A15

Optimised Treatment Modalities for Hypoxic Tumour Cells

P. Workman

MRC Clinical Oncology and Radiotherapeutics Unit, MRC Centre, Hills Road, Cambridge, United Kingdom

Introduction

Solid tumours are made up of many different cell types, including heterogeneous neoplastic subpopulations. The targeting of therapeutic strategies to particular cell populations within tumours has therefore a sound rational basis. Considerable evidence supports the existence of hypoxic cells in solid tumours, and their role in limiting response to radiotherapy and chemotherapy [1,2].

Biology and Biochemistry of Hypoxia

Hypoxic cells are those existing at an intermediate oxygen tension between well-oxygenated cells (oxic population) and those with insufficient oxygen to support viability (anoxic population). Figure 1 illustrates the two known types of tumour hypoxia. Chronic hypoxia arises when solid tumours outgrow their supportive vasculature. This is the classic model of tumour hypoxia [1,3]. The diffusion distance of molecular oxygen is limited by metabolic consumption to 150-200 µm from the nearest capillary. Cells further away from the capillary will become anoxic and non-viable. Those at an intermediate oxygen tension between these cells and the oxic viable population are hypoxic but nevertheless viable. Chronically hypoxic cells have diffusion-limited hypoxia. They are also likely to be starved of nutrients such as glucose, and to accumulate catabolites such as lactic acid.

The second type of hypoxia is acute hypoxia. This is caused by intermittent opening and closing of blood vessels, producing a local and more transient shortage of oxygen [1,4]. Acutely hypoxic cells suffer from perfusion-limited hypoxia, and the time-scale for a given micro-region of tumour to remain hypoxic is likely to be minutes rather than hours or more, in contrast to chronic hypoxia.

Therapeutic Resistance of Hypoxic Cells

Hypoxic cells are 2-3 times more resistant to cell killing by radiation compared to oxic cells [15]. The oxygen tension at which cells display sensitivity midway between those in nitrogen and those in air or pure oxygen is around 0.5% (Km value). This phenomenon is known as the oxygen effect. It arises because molecular oxygen is able to interact with radiation-induced radicals in DNA, leading to irreversible fixation of the damage [2,5]. According to the radiochemical competition model, molecular oxygen competes with reducing species, e.g. thiols such as glutathione, which are able to restore the target molecule to the original undamaged form [5].

Hypoxic cells are also resistant to some chemotherapeutic drugs, including for example bleomycin and some alkylating agents [6]. This may arise through impaired drug delivery, the induction of a non-cycling cell kinetic status or the involvement of molecular oxygen in the mechanism of action of the drug. Recent work has shown that exposure to hypoxia

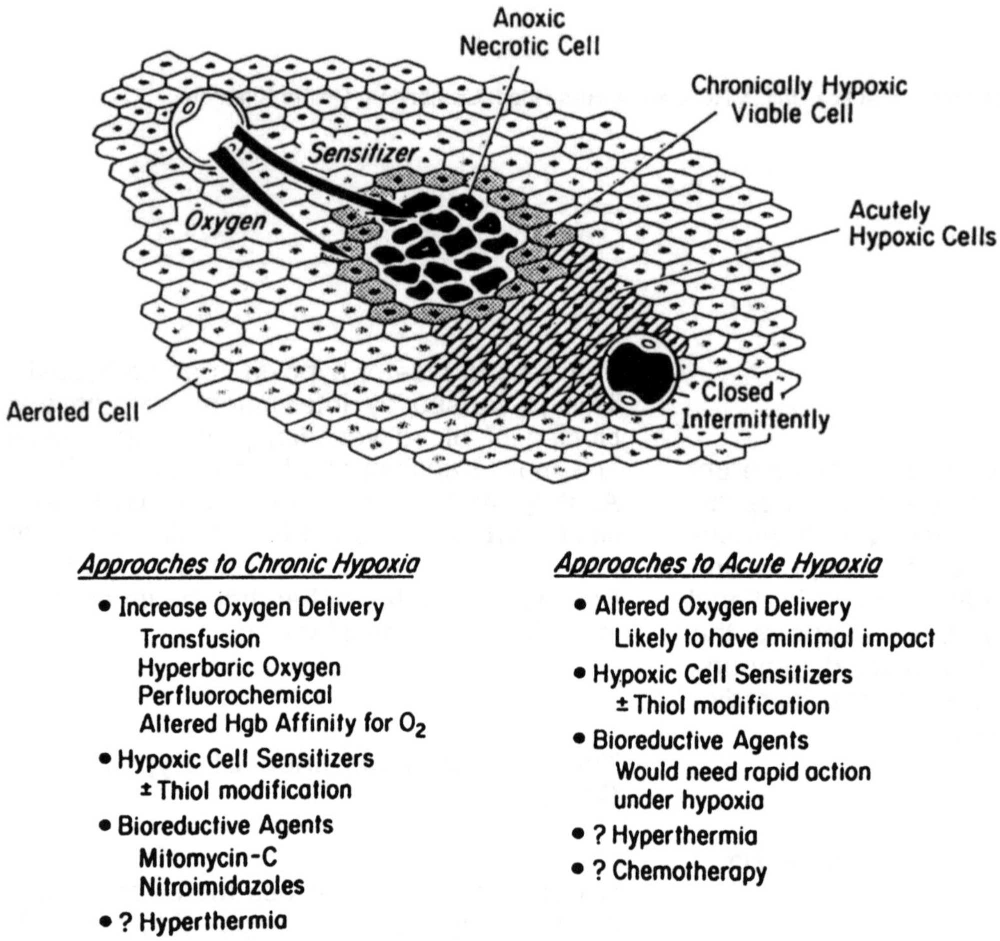

Fig. 1. Chronic and acute hypoxia: possible therapeutic strategies. Reproduced with permission from Coleman [1]

leads to the cellular expression of new proteins, the so-called oxygen-regulated proteins [7]. Relatively transient hypoxia can lead to an enhanced frequency of dihydrofolate reductase gene amplification and hence to methotrexate resistance [8].

Treatment of Hypoxic Tumour Cells

Rational therapies devised to deal with hypoxic tumour cells will involve the combination of hypoxic cell-targeted strategies alongside those aimed to eradicate the oxic population. This will consist of drug combinations or combined modality treatment.

Different approaches may be used to deal with chronic versus acute hypoxia (Fig. 1). For example, techniques designed to increase oxygen delivery, including hyperbaric oxygen, perfluorochemical carriers, transfusions and haemoglobin-modifying agents, would be expected to have greater utility in chronic hypoxia. On the other hand, hypoxic cell sensitising drugs and thiol modifying agents should be equally efficacious against both acute and chronic hypoxia. Bioreductive drugs have undoubted value against chronically hypoxic cells but would probably need to undergo particularly rapid metabolism and reaction to have activity against acutely hypoxic cells.

Recent Advances

The scope of this brief review is to describe some recent advances in the following areas: 1) Improved techniques for the identification and quantitation of hypoxic tumour cells; 2) Development of improved nitroimidazole radiosensitisers; 3) Development of improved nitroimidazole chemosensitisers; 4) Development of improved bioreductive drugs; 5) Manipulation of tissue hypoxia; 6) Role of thiol depletion; 7) Flow cytometry for analysis of biochemical heterogeneity.
Emphasis will be on examples taken from the author's laboratory.

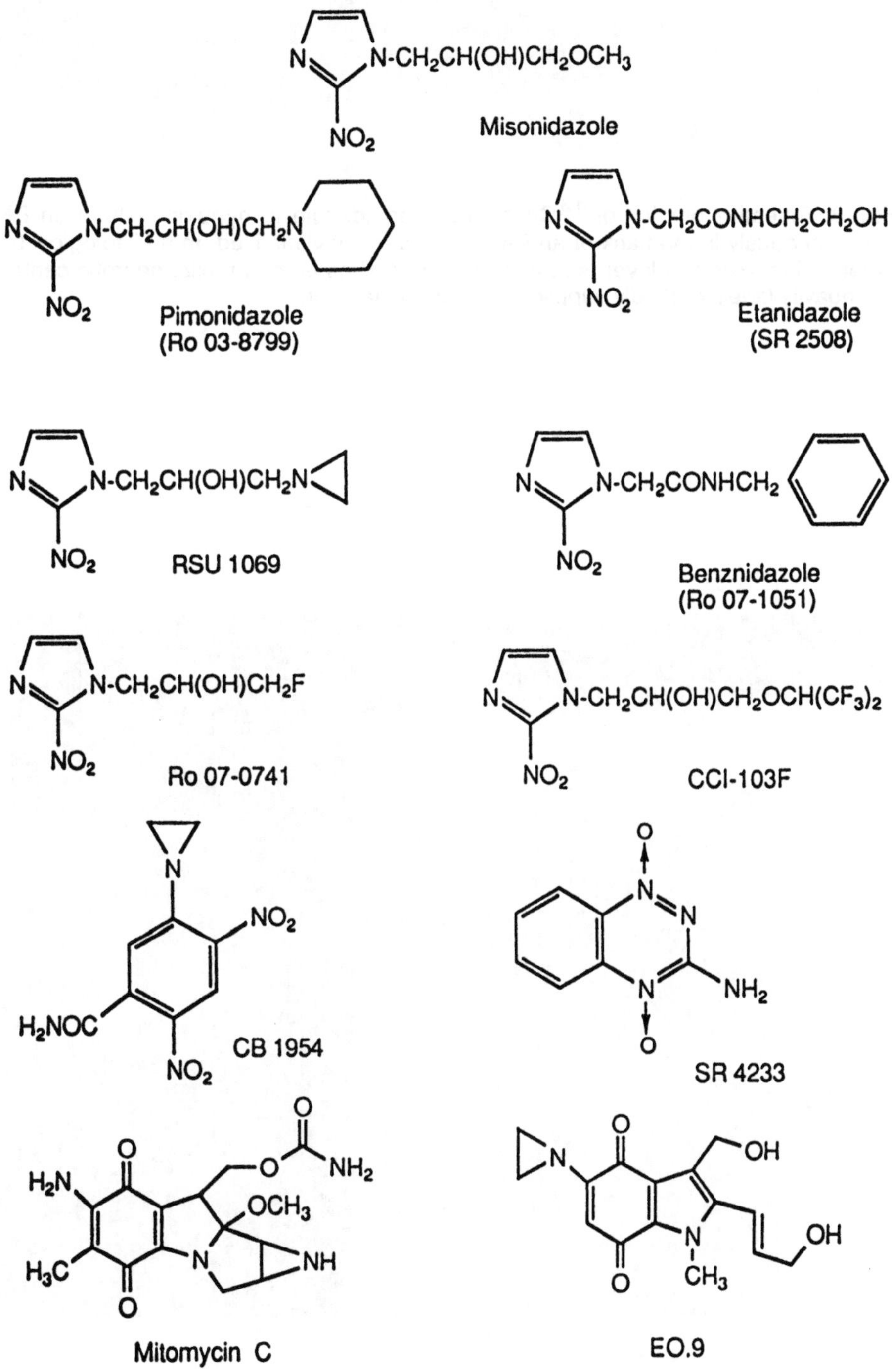

Fig. 2. Chemical structures of some hypoxic cell sensitisers, cytotoxins and hypoxia markers

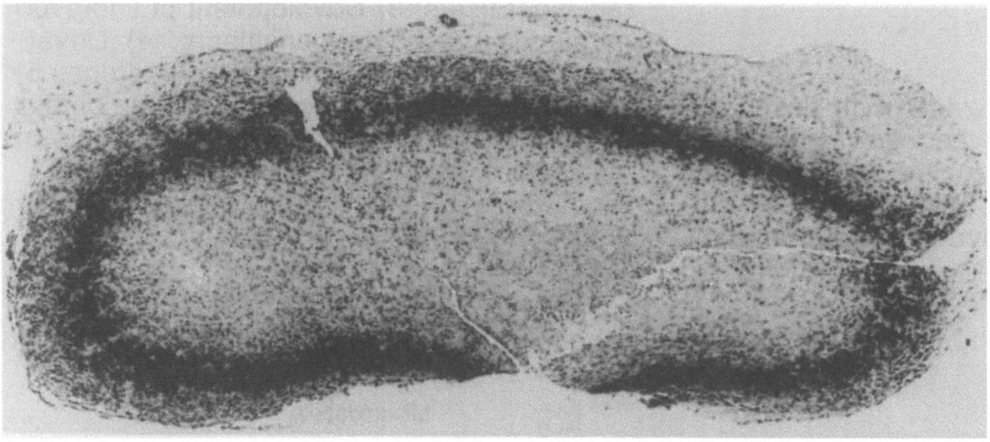

Fig. 3. Selective binding of ^{14}C-labelled misonidazole to hypoxic cells in an EMT6 mouse mammary tumour grown subcutaneously in the flank of an BALB/c mouse, as visualised on a histological tissue section by autoradiography. The outer viable, oxic cell layer is relatively unstained as is the anoxic, necrotic centre, while the intermediate hypoxic cells are heavily labelled. Kindly supplied by Dr J D Chapman

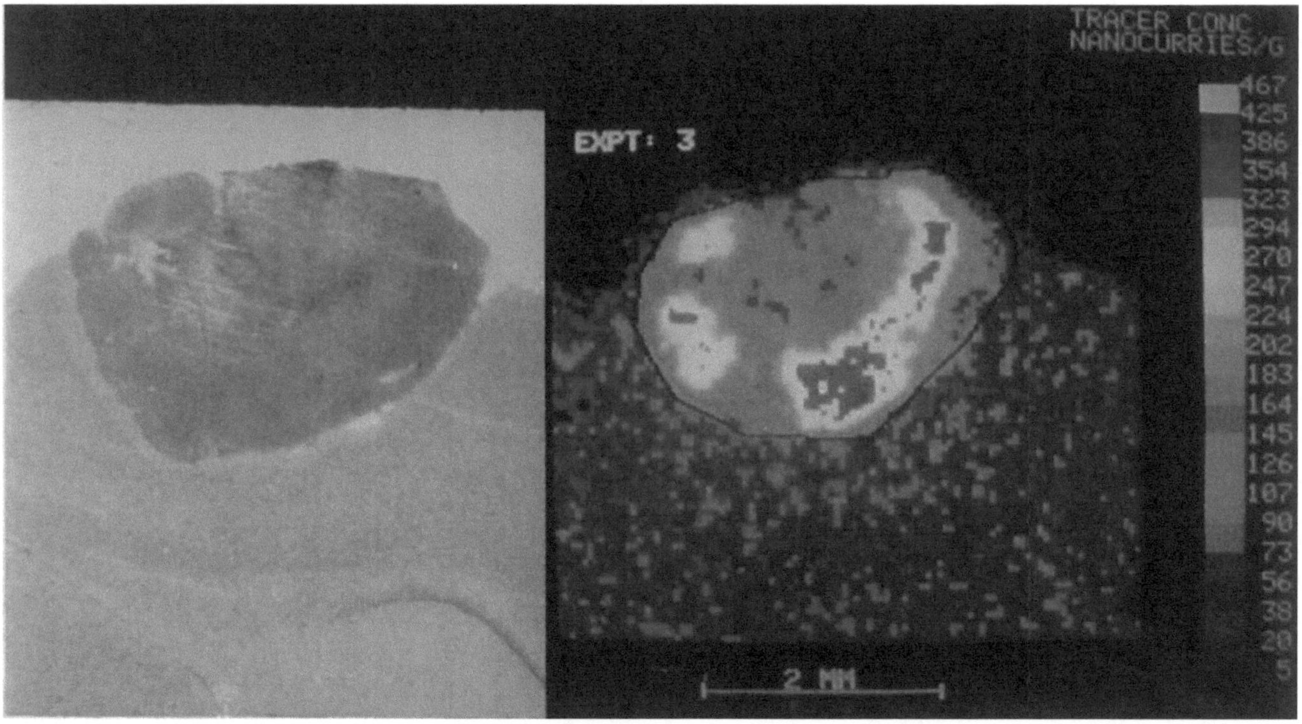

Fig. 4. Left panel: A histological section of rat brain containing an RT-9 brain tumour (H and E stained). Right panel: Quantitative autoradiograph of an adjacent frozen section showing preferential localisation of ^{14}C-misonidazole in the viable region of the tumour close to the necrotic centre. Reproduced with permission from Horowitz et al. [11]

Identifying and Quantifying Tumour Hypoxia

Application of hypoxia-targeted strategies will be made more efficient if patients most likely to benefit could be identified. Pioneering work by Chapman and colleagues [9] showed that the 2-nitroimidazole misonidazole (Fig. 2) can be used in a radiolabelled form to identify and quantify tumour hypoxia. This agent was used in early clinical trials as a radiosensitiser and is still under evaluation as a chemosensitiser [2]. It undergoes bioreductive metabolism at the nitro group under hypoxia leading to binding to nucleic acids and proteins which can be visualised on tissue sections by autoradiography [9,10]. Fig. 3 shows selective labelling of hypoxic cells in an EMT6 mouse mammary tumour grown subcutaneously in the flank of a mouse.

A further elegant demonstration of this technique showed that labelled misonidazole distributed uniformly across the "normal" rat brain at early times after drug administration, but penetration into the experimental RT-9 brain tumour in the same animals showed much greater regional variability [11]. At later times tumour radioactivity levels became much higher than in surrounding "normal" brain and particularly marked retention of label occurred around apparently viable cells located close to necrotic foci (Fig. 4).

In recent clinical studies, tritiated misonidazole binding to potentially hypoxic tumour regions was seen in 2 patients (one small cell lung cancer and one melanoma) out of a total of 6 [12]. This technique is, however, lengthy and laborious and alternative techniques have been sought.

A polyclonal antibody was raised to a hemocyanin adduct of a reductively activated, hexafluorinated analogue of misonidazole CCI-103F (Fig. 2). Fluorescence immunohistochemistry showed antibody reactivity towards those regions of spheroids and tumours in which the ^{3}H-labelled drug was located by autoradiography [13]. This technique would avoid the use of radioisotopes but would still be surgically invasive, which is a disadvantage for repeated analysis of the hypoxic fraction, e.g. during fractionated radiotherapy.

Magnetic resonance spectroscopy (MRS) has the advantage that it can be carried out repeatedly and non-invasively on tumours *in situ*. ^{19}F-MRS gives high sensitivity and low background. *In vitro* spectra were obtained for tissues excised from mice given CCI-103F [14]. We subsequently showed [15] that ^{19}F-MRS spectra could be obtained for tumours *in*

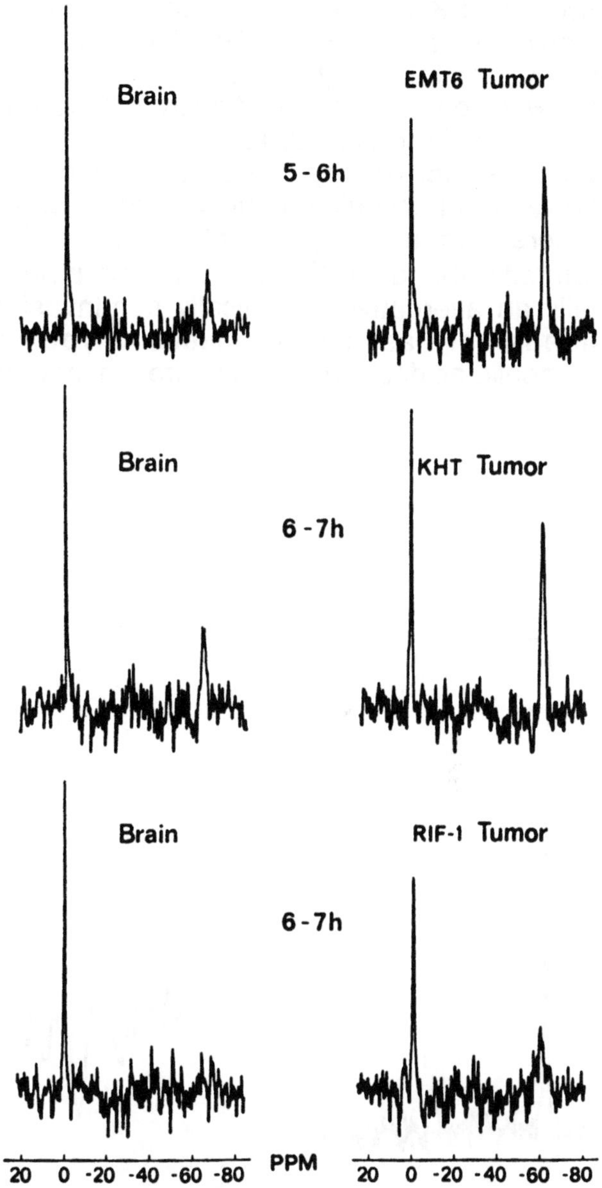

Fig. 5. ^{19}F magnetic resonance spectra of EMT6, KHT and RIF-1 tumours (grown id in the flank) *in vivo* 5-7 h after administration of 2 mmol/kg of monofluorinated misonidazole analogue Ro 07-0741 to BALB/c or C3H/He mice. Spectra were obtained on a 1.9 T Oxford Research Systems TMR-32 spectrometer using a 15 mm surface coil and 900 pulses at a 1 sec pulse repetition time over 15 min. In each case the peak at approx -60 ppm corresponds to Ro 07-0741-related material, while that at 0 ppm is the 5-fluorouracil external shift reference. Peak height is proportional to concentration. Reproduced with permission from Maxwell, Workman and Griffiths [15]

situ using either CCI-103F or the monofluorinated probe Ro 07-0741 (Fig. 2). Whereas MRS signal disposition was uniform at early times, retention of signal was greatest in tumour tissue compared to brain and liver, probably related to bioreductive metabolism and binding. Also, signal was much higher in EMT6 and KHT tumours, which have higher hypoxic fractions, than in RIF-1 which has a low hypoxic fraction (Fig. 5).

We went on to compare directly results obtained for ^{19}F-nitroimidazole probe retention with those for energy charge estimated from the ratio of nucleotide triphosphates or phosphocreatine to inorganic phosphate using naturally abundant ^{31}P-MRS. This is potentially an alternative, chemically non-invasive means of assessing tissue hypoxia. Metabolic acidosis which may predominate in hypoxic regions of tumours can also be assessed from the chemical shift in the inorganic phosphate resonance. ^{19}F and ^{31}P spectra for the same EMT6 tumour are shown in Fig. 6. In fact, the results showed the ^{31}P spectra to be highly heterogeneous between tumours. In addition, a small hypoxic population would most likely be masked by the more abundant oxic population. Thus, unless very marked hypoxia is anticipated, there is likely to be a real advantage for probes such as the ^{19}F-nitroimidazoles which are specific for the minority hypoxic population.

It should be mentioned that the magnetic field used in these experiments was similar to those available on whole-body magnetic resonance imaging machines: thus MRS imaging of hypoxic cells may become feasible.

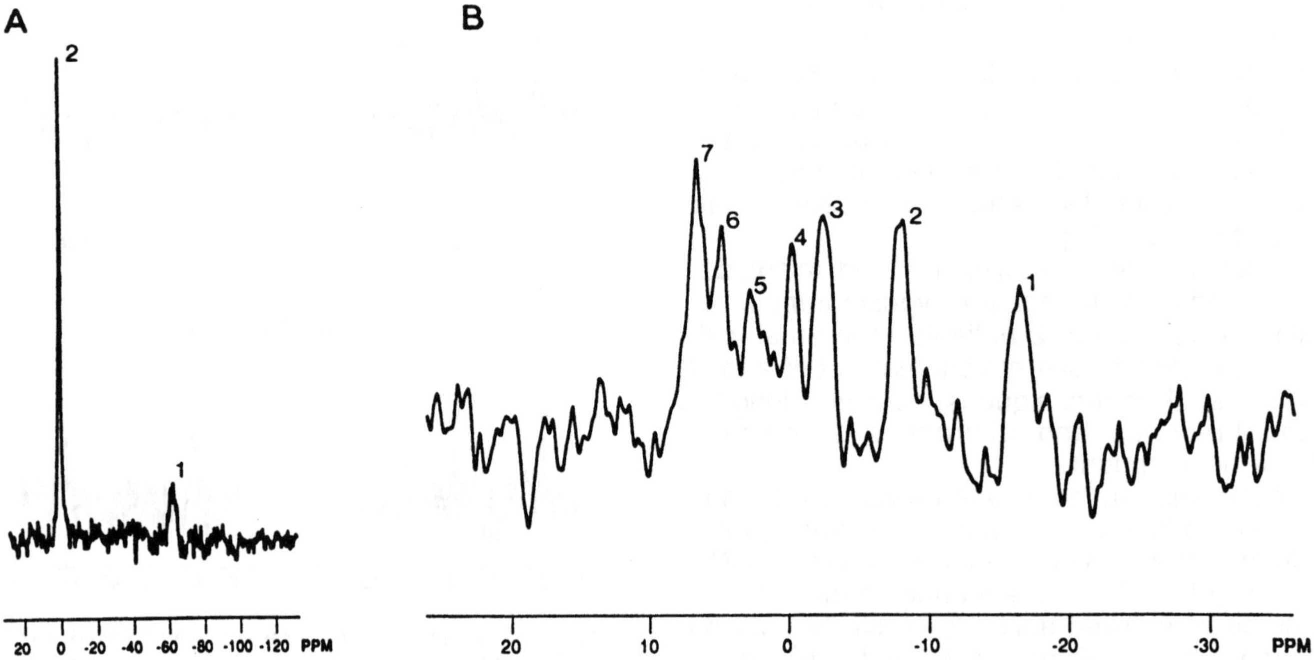

Fig. 6. A. ^{19}F magnetic resonance spectrum of an EMT6 tumour *in vivo* 20 h after administration of 2 mmol/kg Ro 07-0741 to a BALB/c mouse. Peak assignments: 1, Ro 07-0741-related material; 2, 5-fluorouracil external shift reference. **B.** ^{31}P magnetic resonance spectrum of the same tumour shortly before administration of Ro 07-0741. Peak assignments are: 1, beta-phosphate of nucleoside triphosphates (NTP); 2, alpha-phosphate of NTP; 3, gamma-phosphate of NTP; 4, phosphocreatine; 5, phosphodiesters; 6, inorganic phosphate; 7, phosphomonoesters. Other details were as in Fig. 5.
Data from Workman, P, Maxwell R J and Griffiths J R (unpublished)

Development of Improved Nitroimidazole Radiosensitisers

Electron-affinic nitroheterocyclic compounds are able to sensitise hypoxic cells to radiation damage via a fast free radical mechanism analogous to that for molecular oxygen [2,5]. Thus, their activity is "oxygen-mimetic". Radiosensitisation efficiency is primarily a function of the ease with which the nitro group is able to accept an electron. This "electron affinity" is measured by the one-electron reduction potential.

However, whereas the radiosensitisation mechanism for these agents is identical to that for molecular oxygen, the active nitro group can be delivered to hypoxic cells more efficiently because of slower metabolic consumption. Pharmacokinetics and tissue disposition can be modulated by modifying the side-chain substituents.

Misonidazole showed excellent penetration into human tumours but extensive evaluation showed that doses were limited by peripheral and central neurotoxicity [16]. This experience had a negative influence on the continued development of hypoxic cell sensitisers [17].

The development of the 2 new analogues currently undergoing clinical trial was based primarily on the concept of optimising peak tumour sensitiser levels during radiotherapy while minimising systemic exposure (Fig. 7). The essential features for pimonidazole and etanidazole are summarised in Fig. 8.

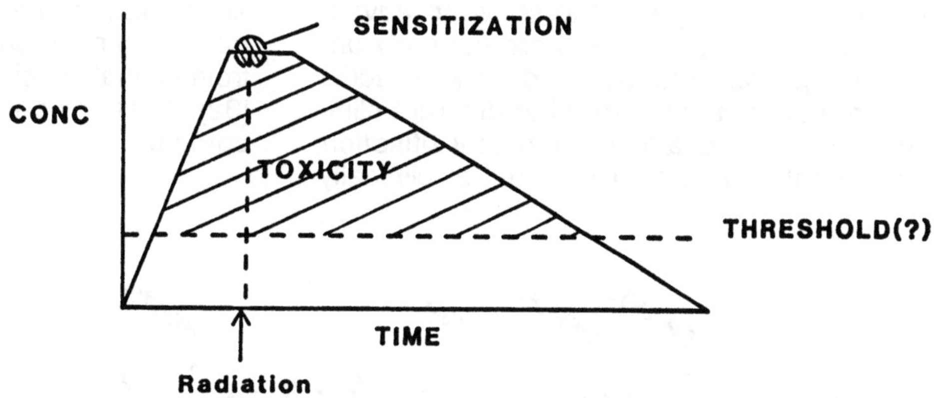

Fig. 7. Concept underlying the design of improved radiosensitisers. Sensitisation is related to tumour concentration during radiation, while neurotoxicity is a function of systemic and particularly nervous tissue exposure. Reproduced with permission from Workman [18]

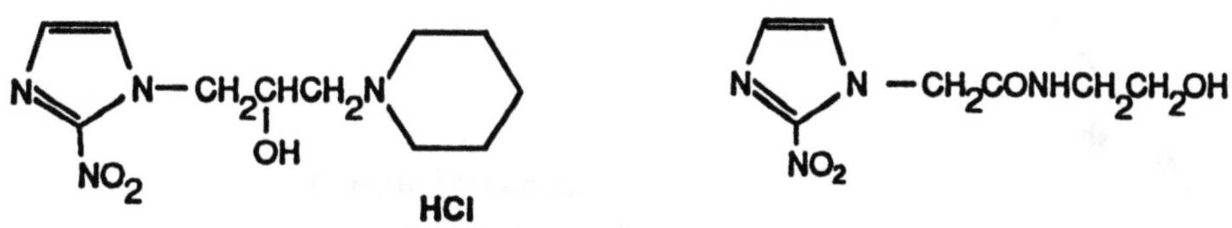

Pimonidazole (Ro 03-8799)

- Lipophilic free base, extensively protonated
- More potent radiosensitization than misonidazole
- Rapid accumulation in brain and peripheral nerve
- Metabolic and renal clearance
- Acute CNS syndrome limits individual doses to 0.75-1 g/m²; no peripheral neuropathy

Etanidazole (SR 2508)

- Hydrophilic, neutral
- Equal radiosensitization potency to misonidazole
- Slow uptake into brain and peripheral nerve
- Renal clearance
- Peripheral neuropathy limits total dose to 36-40 g/m²; no acute CNS syndrome

Fig. 8. Important features of pimonidazole and etanidazole in relation to their development as improved radiosensitisers. Reproduced with permission from Workman [19]

Etanidazole has the major advantage of relative exclusion from brain and peripheral nerve, as predicted from its hydrophilic character (Fig. 9). Clinical studies showed etanidazole to be excluded from human brain but not tumour tissue as a result of the breakdown of the blood-brain barrier (Fig. 10). Although peripheral neuropathy is still seen, the drug can be given at 3 times the total dose for misonidazole [22].

The basicity of pimonidazole was expected to lead to its rapid elimination in acid urine. In fact, a major feature is its accumulation in cells [23] and tissue [21,24], and also its affinity for DNA [25]. Fig. 10 shows how pimonidazole accumulates in both normal brain and brain tumour tissue. Peripheral neuropathy is not seen but an acute CNS syndrome is dose-limiting [26,27].

Both drugs are expected to show an advantage over misonidazole and are currently undergoing phase III randomised trials. In addition, in view of their somewhat different clinical toxicities and additive radiosensitisation demonstrated in a mouse model at clinically relevant tumour concentrations [28], clinical studies with the two drugs in combination are also ongoing [21,29]. Although some interactive toxicity is seen, the combination appears promising with respect to either agent alone.

Completing the series of lead compounds in current radiosensitiser development is the analogue RSU 1069 (Fig. 12). This is a mixed-function analogue containing both an electron-affinic nitro group and an alkylating aziridine moiety. It shows highly potent radiosensitisation of hypoxic cells *in vitro* and *in vivo* [30] through its ability to be targeted to DNA, where bioreduction can generate a cross-linking species.

Preclinical pharmacokinetic behaviour was acceptable [31]. Though some scope for fine-tuning of neoplastic tissue penetration was identified for some transplantable tumours, accumulation was seen in others. Unfortunately, clinical trials revealed severe gastrointestinal toxicity at relatively modest doses [32]. Less toxic analogues are under development.

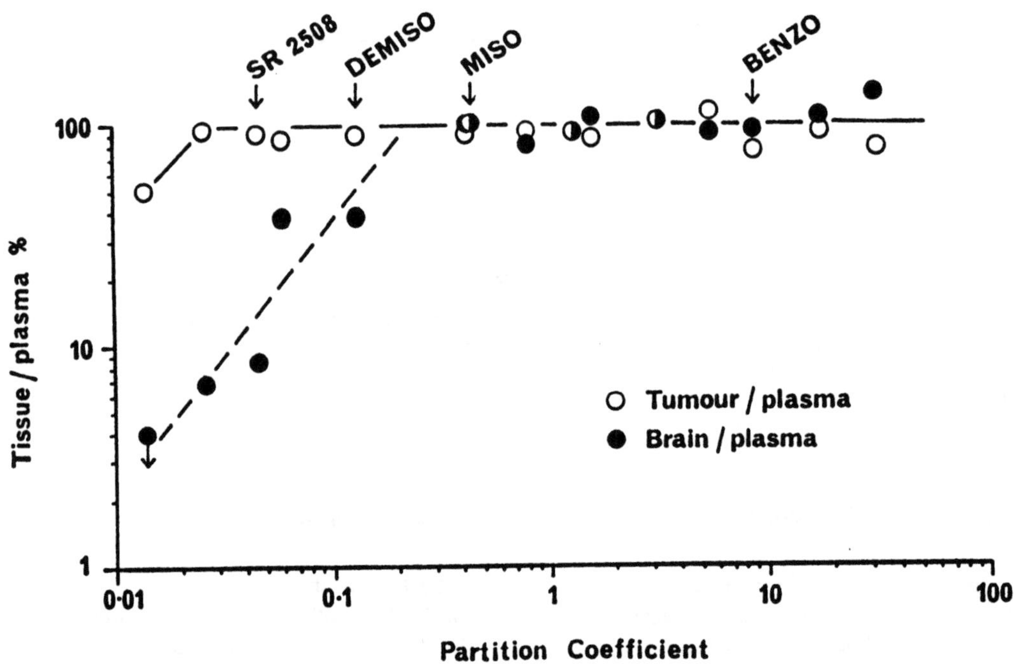

Fig. 9. Lipophilicity-dependent penetration of neutral nitroimidazoles into brain and EMT6 tumour in BALB/c mice. Ratios were averaged over 20-135 min. Abbreviations: SR 2508, etanidazole; DEMISO, desmethylmisonidazole; MISO, misonidazole; BENZO, benznidazole. Redrawn with permission from Brown and Workman [3] with additional data from the author

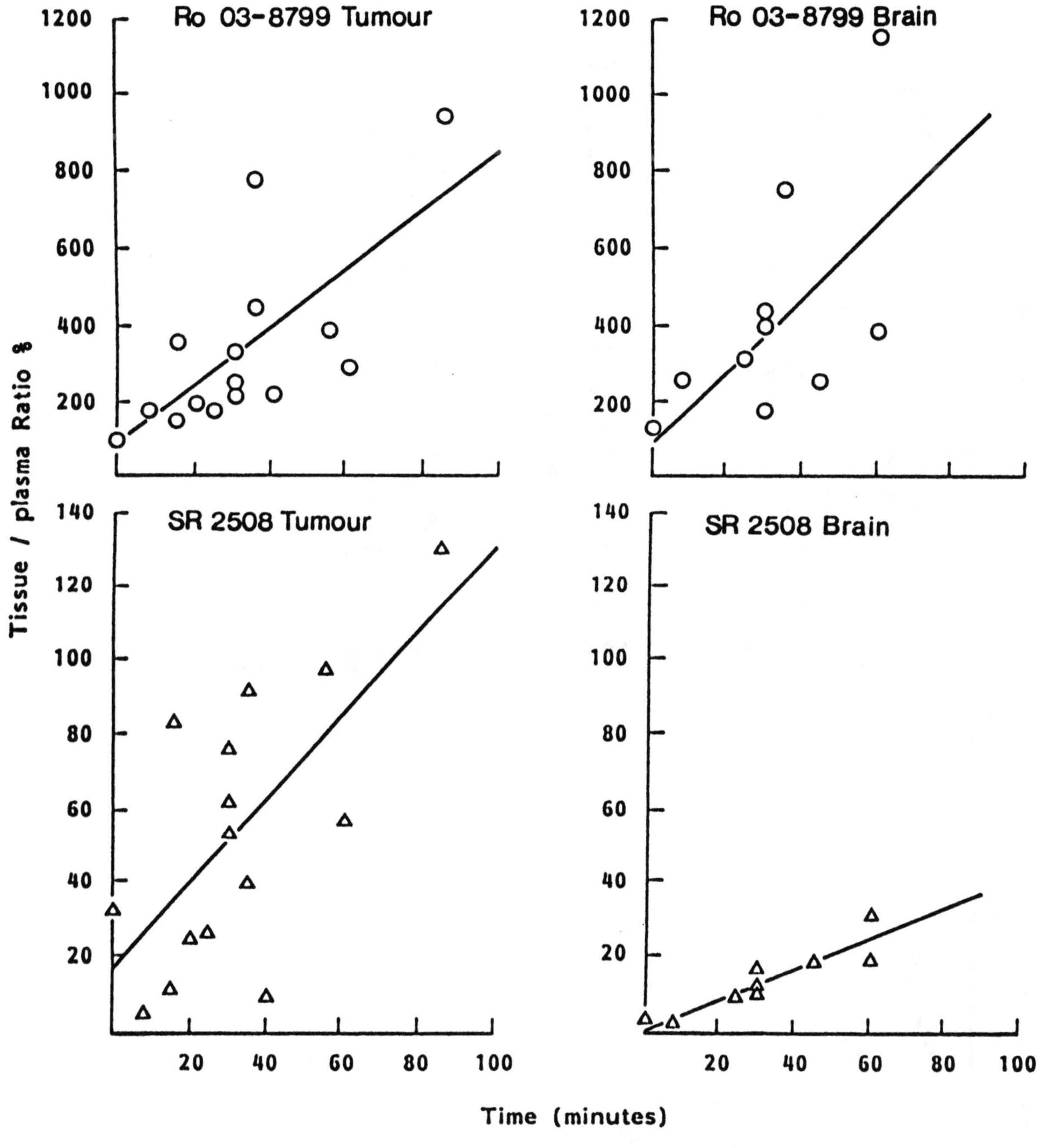

Fig. 10. Differential penetration of etanidazole and pimonidazole into brain tumour and adjacent normal brain of patients, plotted as a function of time after the end of infusion of the combination. Reproduced with permission from Newman et al. [21]

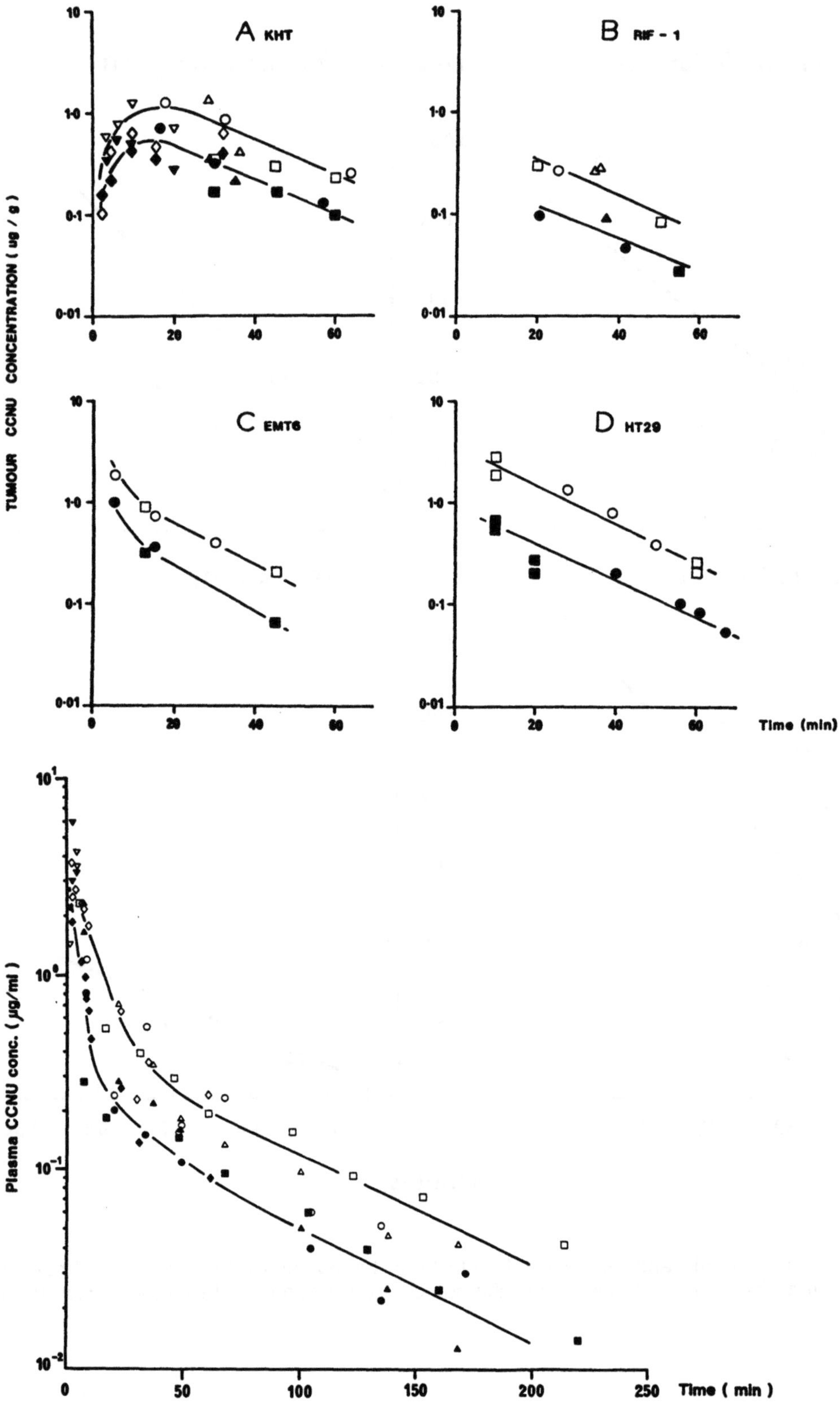

Fig. 11. Effects of misonidazole (2.5 mmol/kg ip) on the plasma pharmacokinetics and tumour disposition of CCNU (20 mg/kg ip) in C3H mice. Above: uptake of CCNU into the KHT (A) and RIF-1 (B) sarcomas grown im in C3H/He mice, the EMT6 mouse mammary tumour im in BALB/c mice (C) and the HT29 human colon adenocarcinoma xenograft sc in CBA nude mice (D). Below: plasma pharmacokinetics of CCNU.
Open symbols indicate CCNU was given 30 min after misonidazole; closed symbols indicate CCNU after misonidazole vehicle as control. Reproduced with permission from Lee and Workman [41]

Development of Improved Nitroimidazole Chemosensitisers

Misonidazole was identified to have the ability to sensitise hypoxic cells to certain chemotherapeutic agents, particularly alkylating agents and chloroethylnitrosoureas [33,34]. A large number of studies were carried out in animals, and there was some controversy over whether misonidazole exhibited activity at clinically relevant sensitiser concentrations.

This led to the search for improved chemosensitisers compared to misonidazole. Although none showed a greater effect than misonidazole at high sensitiser doses, the mixed-function compound RSU 1069 and the lipophilic analogue benznidazole (Fig. 2) both exhibited more potent activity [30,35]. A comparison of their activities with respect to CCNU chemosensitisation is shown in Table 1.

A phase I clinical trial of benznidazole [36] showed that exposures could be achieved in man which generate significant sensitisation of CCNU response in mice. However, results of a phase II study of benznidazole with CCNU in melanoma [37] and a phase III study in glioma [38] revealed no major advantage over CCNU alone.

In the meantime the results of a randomised phase II trial of melphalan with or without misonidazole for non-small cell lung cancer has demonstrated benefit for the sensitiser [39]. Because of the higher sensitiser doses which can be given, clinical studies with etanidazole combined with cyclosphosphamide are now in progress.

Studies on the mechanism of action of chemosensitisation have focused on 2 main areas: 1) alteration in systemic pharmacokinetics and metabolism of the cytotoxic agent and 2) hypoxia-mediated effects at the target tumour cell level [33,40]. Modified pharmacokinetics may well contribute to the chemosensitisation of CCNU by misonidazole and benznidazole. Changes in liver metabolism and plasma pharmacokinetics can lead to a preferential increase in tumour versus normal tissue concentrations, probably as a result of blood flow considerations [41,42]. With oral CCNU in mice altered pharmacokinetics can lead to chemoprotection [43].

Table 1. Dose-modifying factors for chemosensitisation of the response of tumour and normal tissues to lomustine by single doses of nitroimidazoles in C3H/He mice

Sensitiser (mmols/kg)	Investigating group[2]	Dose-modifying factor[1]: Tumour[3] (KHT sarcoma)	Peripheral wbcs [4]	Bone marrow (CFU-S)	Lethality[5] (LD50)
Misonidazole (2.5-5.0)	A	1.8-2.4	1.0		1.2-1.4
	B	1.5	1.0		1.1
	C	1.5-1.9		1.0-1.5	
Benznidazole (0.3)	A	2.0			1.3-1.4
	B	1.5-2.0	1.2		1.3
RSU 1069 (0.38)	A	1.9	1.0		1.0-1.2

1 Isoeffect dose for lomustine alone/isoeffect dose for lomustine plus chemosensitiser. Results are for single doses of sensitiser and lomustine. Drugs were given ip, either simultaneously or with the sensitiser given 30-60 mins before lomustine
2 A = Rochester, NY, B = Cambridge, England, and C = Stanford, CA
3 Regrowth delay or clonogenic survival
4 Day 3 (nadir)
5 30 days
Reproduced with permission from Workman [35]

Detailed studies showed that both misonidazole and particularly benznidazole were able to act as Type II inhibitors of mouse liver microsomal cytochrome P-450 [44] leading to powerful inhibition of CCNU monohydroxylation by this haemoprotein (Fig. 12). A schematic representation of the interaction of benznidazole with cytochrome P-450 is shown in Fig. 13.

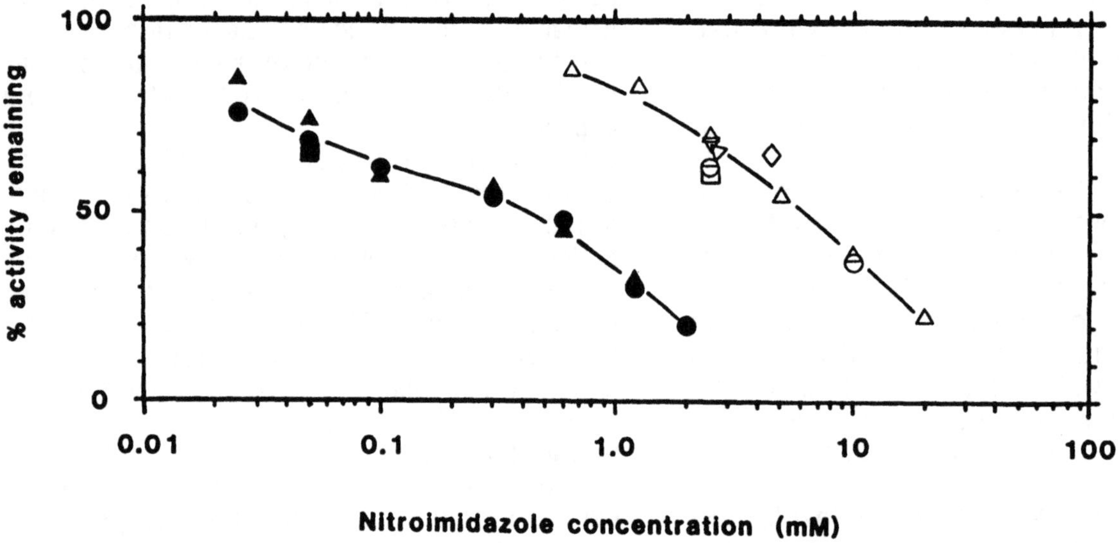

Fig. 12. Inhibition by misonidazole (open symbols) and benznidazole (closed symbols) of CCNU monohydroxylation by C3H mouse liver microsomal cytohrome P-450 *in vitro*. Reproduced with permission from Lee, Workman and Cheeseman [44]

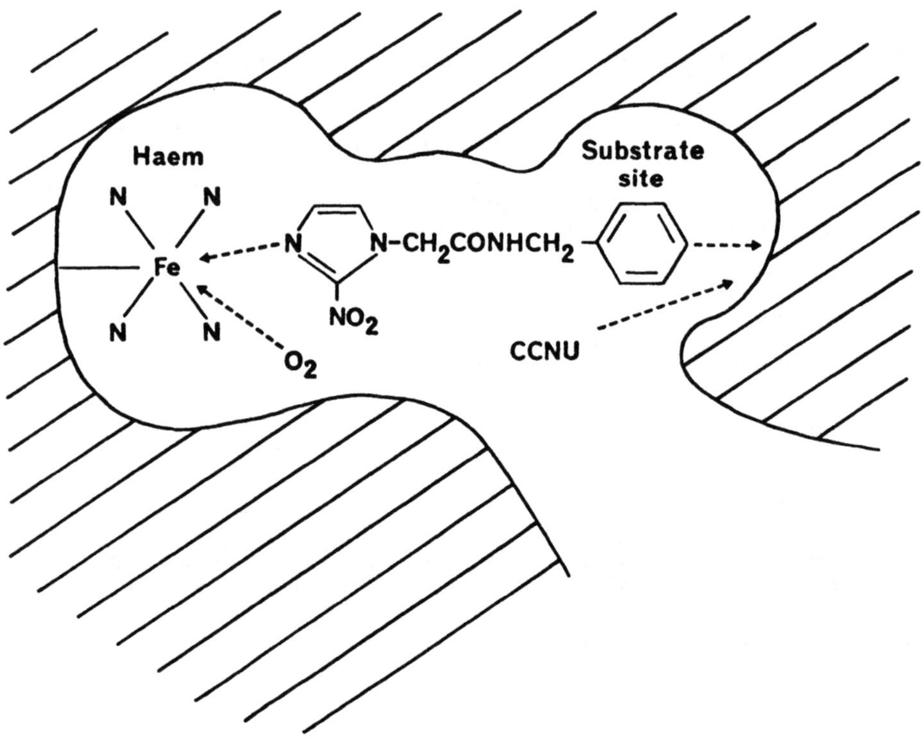

Fig. 13. Schematic representation of the interaction between benznidazole and the active site of cytochrome P-450

Table 2. Relationship between predicted and actual inhibition of CCNU hydroxylation by benznidazole (BENZO) in man

Patient [1]	BENZO dose [2] (mg/kg)	Plasma BENZO [3] at 4h (µg/ml)	Predicted [4] inhibition (%)	Peak CCNU [3] (µg/ml)
A-K	0	0	0	0
L	8	10.4	20	0
M	12	20.5	30	0
N	14	26.9	33	0.02
O	14	25.6	32	0
P	17	25.6	32	0.05
Q	20	39.2	38	0.63
E	25	28.3	34	0.31
F	25	48.7	40	0.44
G	25	28.6	34	0.22
H	25	54.3	41	0.17
I	25	22.8	31	0.062
J	25	41.5	39	0.058
K	25	5.7	15	0
R	25	37.9	38	0.23
S	25	32.4	36	0.12
T	40	63.3	43	0.14
U	40	48.3	40	0.21
V	40	27.9	34	0.24

1 Some patients received both CCNU alone and CCNU with BENZO on separate occasions
2 Given orally 4h before an oral dose of 130 mg/m^2 CCNU
3 By HPLC
4 From Fig. 1
Reproduced with permission from Workman et al. [45]

Clinical studies showed that cytochrome P-450 inhibition occurred in man at similar benznidazole concentrations as were inhibitory *in vitro* and in mice, resulting in the appearance of parent CCNU in the plasma (Table 2).

A pharmacokinetic component was also recognised in the complex interaction between misonidazole and melphalan in mice [46-48]. In addition, a pronounced decrease in structural and functional vascular volume was seen following misonidazole (49). In the case of pharmacokinetic interaction between nitroimidazoles and chloroethylnitrosoureas, both the modifier and the cytotoxic agent must have a certain degree of lipophilicity, making them more likely to interact with hepatic cytochrome P-450 [50]. Thus the pharmacokinetic component of chemosensitisation can be designed out by increasing the hydrophilic character of the nitroimidazole and/or the nitrosourea. No serious pharmacokinetic interaction was seen with misonidazole and melphalan in man [40] and such effects are even less likely with the more hydrophilic sensitisers such as etanidazole.

Although local and/or systemic changes in the handling of the cytotoxic drug can be very important, it is clear that there is a quite different and much more specific mechanism operating at the level of the hypoxic cell [33,40]. Requirements for the absence of oxygen are quite rigorous, with maximum chemosensitisation requiring as little as 0.05% - 0.5% oxygen. This implicates the involvement of bioreductive metabolism, and depletion of glutathione is also thought to play a role (see later).

Development of Improved Bioreductive Drugs

The so-called bioreductive drugs exhibit selective cytotoxicity towards hypoxic cells compared to their oxic counterparts, as a result of preferential reductive metabolism to toxic species at very low oxygen levels. They therefore represent a special class of enzyme-activated prodrugs. In general the toxic species are thought to exert their effects through reaction with DNA and protein in the target cell.

Until recently the main classes of bioreductive antitumour agents have been the nitro compounds such as misonidazole and quinone type agents exemplified by mitomycin C (Fig. 2) [51]. A highly promising new class, the benzotriazine di-N-oxides such as SR 4233 (Fig. 2), has now been introduced as well [52]. Although the requirement for metabolic activation has been well recognised, the importance of defining the participation of individual reductases and their regulatory control has not been so well appreciated. Multiple reductases are known to catalyse bioreductive drug activation at low oxygen tension, but the precise role of any one enzyme for a given reaction is often not known. Bioreduction is often a complex multistep process, and the extent to which different intermediates are formed may well be critical, representing a balance between toxication and detoxication pathways. This will represent the main focus of the present section.

Toxicology and delivery considerations have generally indicated the desirability of maintaining the nitro group within a heterocyclic nucleus, and the 2-nitroimidazoles may be optimal in this respect. Fig. 14 gives a general idea of the complexity of the enzymatic bioreduction of nitro compounds. Firstly, bioreduction involves a multistep sequence of reactions, the important metabolites being the nitro radical anion (1 electron addition), nitroso (2 electrons) and hydroxylamine (4 electrons), all of which are likely to be toxic, while the amine (6 electrons) is regarded as non-toxic. Secondly, multiple enzymes are involved, both soluble and membrane-bound, and each may play a different role at specific parts of the metabolic activation pathway. Thirdly, the picture may well be quite different for each individual agent. Lastly, it may also vary for each tissue or tumour concerned.

Fig. 14 also illustrates the important role of molecular oxygen in controlling the rate of bioreductive activation. Under well-oxygenated conditions, reoxidation of the nitro anion radical to the parent compound occurs with the generation of superoxide. Although this may lead to lipid peroxidation and toxicity in aerobic cells, this is a considerably less toxic pathway than further nitroreduction.

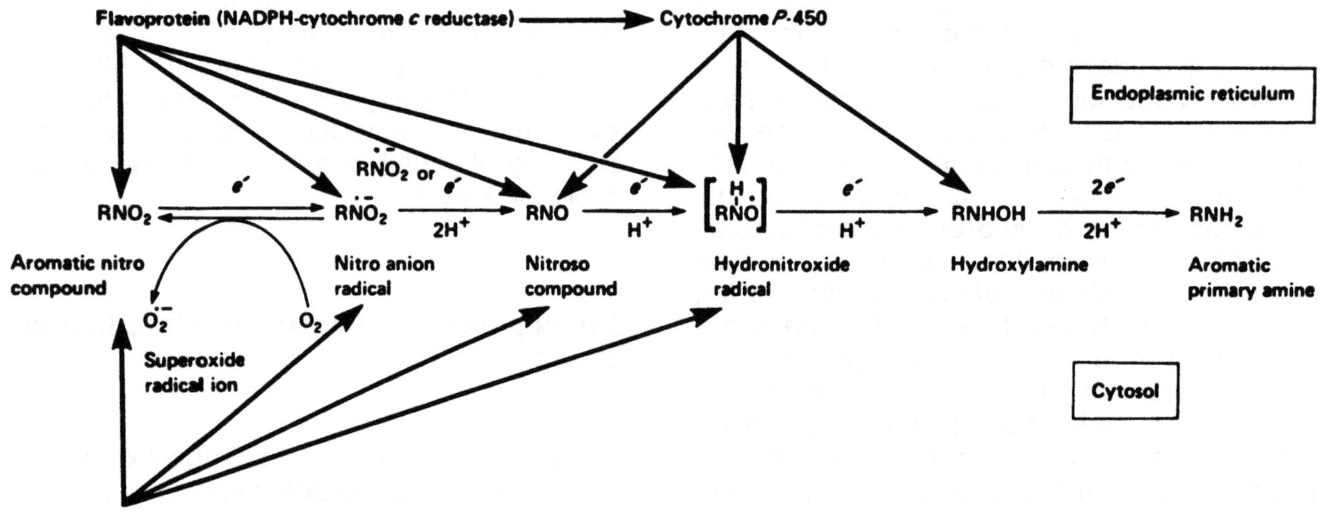

Fig. 14. Schematic illustrating the multistep, multienzyme character of nitroreductive bioactivation pathways. Reproduced with permission from Hewick [53]

We have studied the enzymology of benznidazole bioreduction in particular detail during its development as a chemosensitiser. In mouse liver microsomes, the initial steps are catalysed by cytochrome P-450 reductase, while cytochrome P-450 is preferentially involved at later stages leading to amine formation [53,54]. The predominant role of P-450 reductase in the early stages was confirmed with the purified rat liver enzyme and a specific inhibitory antibody raised against it. P-450 reductase has also been shown to catalyse the reduction of misonidazole [56].

The molecular enzymology of the reductive bioactivation of the dinitrophenyl aziridine CB 1954 (Fig. 2) is extremely interesting. Here, P-450 reductase apparently catalysed reduction more efficiently at the 4-nitro versus the 2-nitro position [55]. The two respective hydroxylamines have been identified and measured by HPLC and their different stabilities may contribute to this apparent difference. Other recent results suggest that the preferential bioreductive activation of CB 1954 to the 4-hydroxylamine by the oxygen-insensitive cytosolic enzyme DT-diaphorase, also known as quinone reductase, may account for the unique susceptibility of the rat Walker tumour to the drug under aerobic conditions [57]. Ongoing studies in our laboratory suggest that multiple additional metabolites may be formed, and that the reaction kinetics are extremely complex under anoxia (Walton MI and Workman P, unpublished).

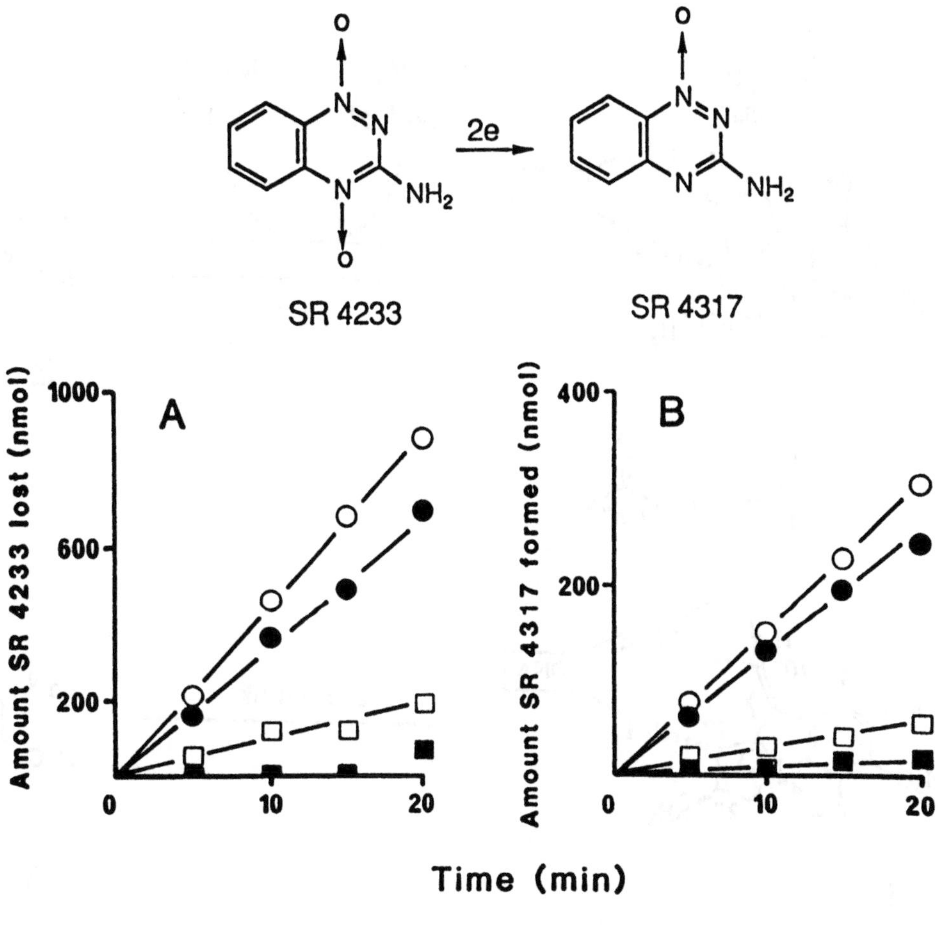

Fig. 15. Bioreductive metabolism of the hypoxic cell cytotoxin SR 4233 to the single N-oxide metabolite SR 4317 by C3H/He mouse liver microsomes *in vitro*. Parent drug loss (A) and metabolite formation (B) were measured simultaneously by HPLC.
○ control; ● plus inhibitory antibody to cytochrome P-450 reductase; □ plus the cytochrome P-450 inhibitor carbon monoxide; ■ plus both inhibitors. The results show that cytochrome P-450 has a more predominant role than P-450 reductase in the reaction mechanism. Data from Walton, Wolfe and Workman [54]

Recent data such as those shown in Fig. 15 have also clarified the role of liver cytochrome P-450 and P-450 reductase in the metabolism of the novel benzotriazine di-N-oxide hypoxic cell cytotoxin SR 4233. This is of interest because of its impressively high preferential toxicity for hypoxic versus oxic cells [52]. An inhibitory antibody to cytochrome P-450 reductase results in only a modest inhibition of SR 4233 loss and SR 4317 formation, while a much greater effect is seen with the cytochrome P-450 inhibitor carbon monoxide. The results support a predominant role for cytochrome P-450 in the reduction mechanism.

In vivo experiments with SR 4233 have shown extensive bioreductive metabolism to SR 4317 and the parent benzotriazine SR 4330 in various mouse tumours, normal liver and, surprisingly, normal brain [58]. Among the various tumours studied, reduction was particularly extensive in the EMT6 mouse mammary tumour.

The precise mechanism of action of SR 4233 is unknown but the existence of a DNA-damaging oxidising radical has been proposed, and the protonated form of the radical N-oxide anion may cleave to generate hydroxyl radicals [59,60]. It is therefore possible that 1 electron addition represents the major bioactivation pathway, while simultaneous addition of 2 electrons generating the single N-oxide SR 4317 is a detoxification route.

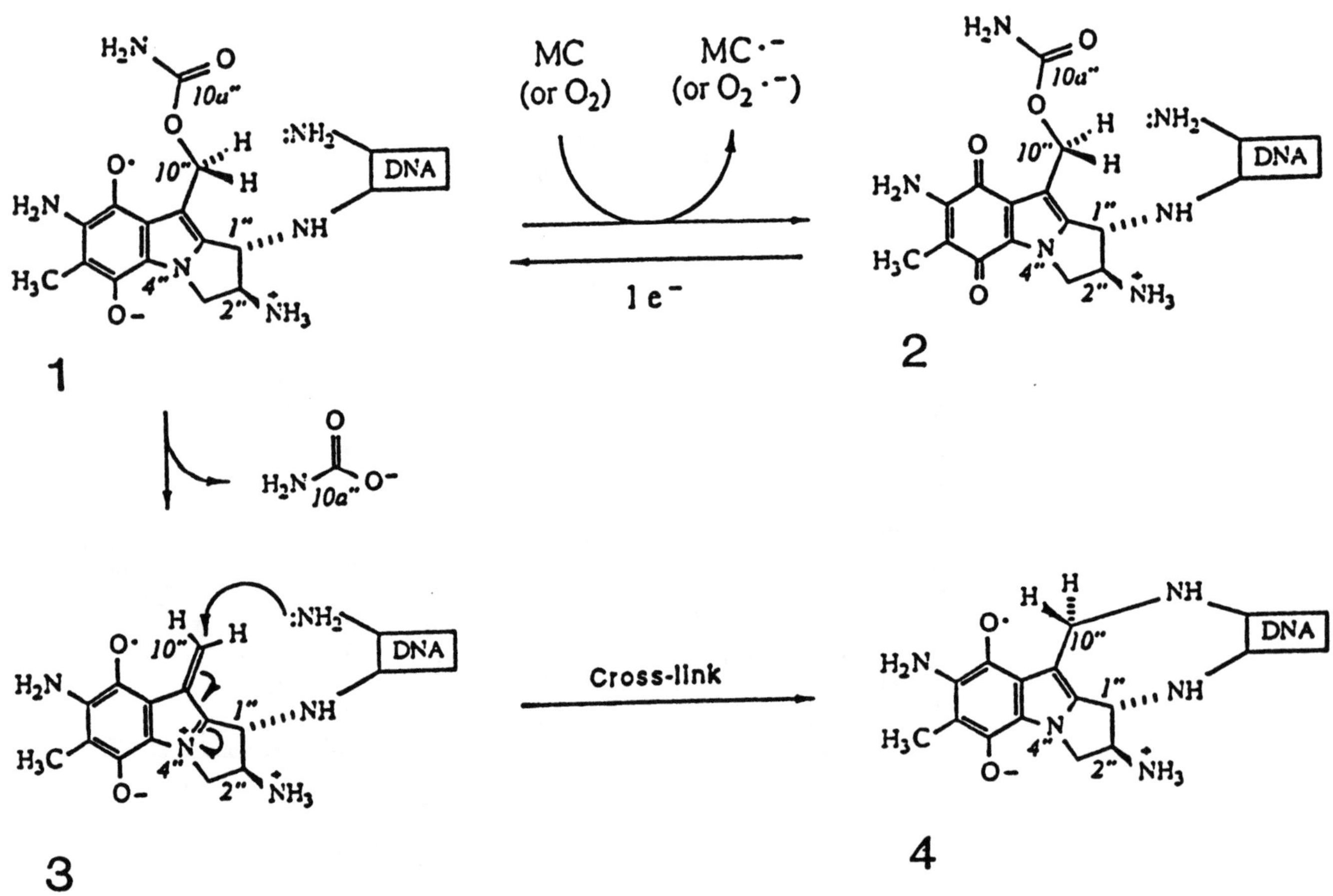

Fig. 16. Mechanism of DNA cross-linking by mitomycin C. The activated mono-adduct formed between C-1 of mitomycin C and guanine N-2 in DNA (structure 1) can react in two ways: in the presence of excess mitomycin C or molecular oxygen formation of the cross-link incompetent quinone mono-adduct (structure 2) is favoured; in the absence of these reactants, carbamate is expelled to produce the iminium species (structure 3) which reacts via C-10 to a neighbouring guanine N-2 forming the cross-link adduct (structure 4). Reproduced with minor modification with permission from Tomasz et al. [63]

Similar to the above scenario, reduction to the semiquinone free radical is thought to be of major importance for the selective hypoxic cell cytotoxicity of the quinone bioreductive agents, while 2 electron reduction to the hydroquinone may be protective [61]. Mitomycin C reacts covalently with DNA following reductive metabolism [51,62,63]. Formation of the semiquinone activates the C-1 position of the aziridine ring and results in alkylation of the N-2 position of guanine in DNA. Subsequent loss of the carbamate side-chain leads to formation of an additional reactive site at C-10, which then alkylates at a second neighbouring guanine N-2 forming a bis-adduct. In this way both intra-strand and inter-strand crosslinks can be formed. Monoadducts can also occur depending on the kinetics of the reaction as shown in Fig. 16.

Computer graphics modelling of the bis-adduct in ß-DNA indicated a snug fit into the minor groove with minimal distortion of the helix, possibly leading to difficulty in damage recognition and repair [63].

Enzymes involved in reductive metabolism of mitomycin C include xanthine oxidase and, more importanly, P-450 reductase which forms the semiquinone free radical [50,62]. Because activated mitomycin C is so reactive with a half-life of around 100 µs and a diffusion distance of about 0.6 µm, nuclear bioreduction may be particularly important [51].

In support of a role for P-450 reductase as a major bioactivating enzyme for mitomycin C, recent results have shown that Chinese hamster ovary cells with acquired resistance to the drug exhibit a marked reduction in expression of this enzyme (Hoban PR, Walton MI, Workman P, Robson CN, Hickson ID and Harris AL, unpublished).

The DT diaphorase inhibitor dicoumarol was found to enhance both the activation of mitomycin C and its cytotoxicity in hypoxic tumour cells, but to reduce toxicity towards oxic cells. This suggested that the DT diaphorase acted as an obligate 2-electron donor leading to detoxication in hypoxic cells, and that inhibition of this pathway facilitated 1-electron bioactivation via 1-electron donors such as cytochrome P-450 reductase. However, it now appears that mitomycin C is unable to act as a substrate for human kidney DT diaphorase [67]. Dicoumarol may therefore modulate mitomycin C cytotoxicity via a different mechanism.

Although it is one of the most widely known bioreductive drugs, mitomycin C in fact exhibits only a modest preferential toxicity towards hypoxic cells (up to 5-fold) [51]. Substitution of a methyl group into the aziridine ring gives the analogue porfiromycin which has considerably greater hypoxic cell selectivity [68]. Modification of 7-amino group of mitomycin C in BMY25282 leads to a more efficient bioactivation and activity in mitomycin C-resistant cells [69].

E0.9 (Fig. 2) is the lead compound in the indoloquinone series under development by the EORTC. Fig. 17 shows that it exhibits much greater potency than mitomycin C against EMT6 cells under aerobic conditions [70]. We have also shown this agent to be selectively toxic under hypoxic conditions and to undergo rapid reductive metabolism *in vitro* and *in vivo* (Kooistra KL, Walton MI and Workman P, unpublished). The enzymes involved are not yet elucidated.

Bioreductive metabolism of the quinone moiety of adriamycin and related compounds leads to cleavage of the sugar moiety and alkylation of cellular macromolecules [71]. Again, cytochrome P-450 reductase is a major enzyme. The precise contribution of this pathway under hypoxic conditions and of superoxide production at higher oxygen tensions is not at all clear in the complex mechanism of action of the anthracyclines.

An interesting approach to the application of bioreductive cytotoxins involves their use in combination with localised tumour hyperthermia. *In vitro* studies have shown that therapeutic hyperthermia (up to 44° C) can be used to accelerate the rate of benznidazole reductive metabolism by tissue extracts *in vitro* [66] and to drive this bioactivation pathway in mouse tumours *in vivo* [73]. This supports the potential role of hyperthermia in combination with bioreductive agents, particularly the hypoxic cell radiosensitisers.

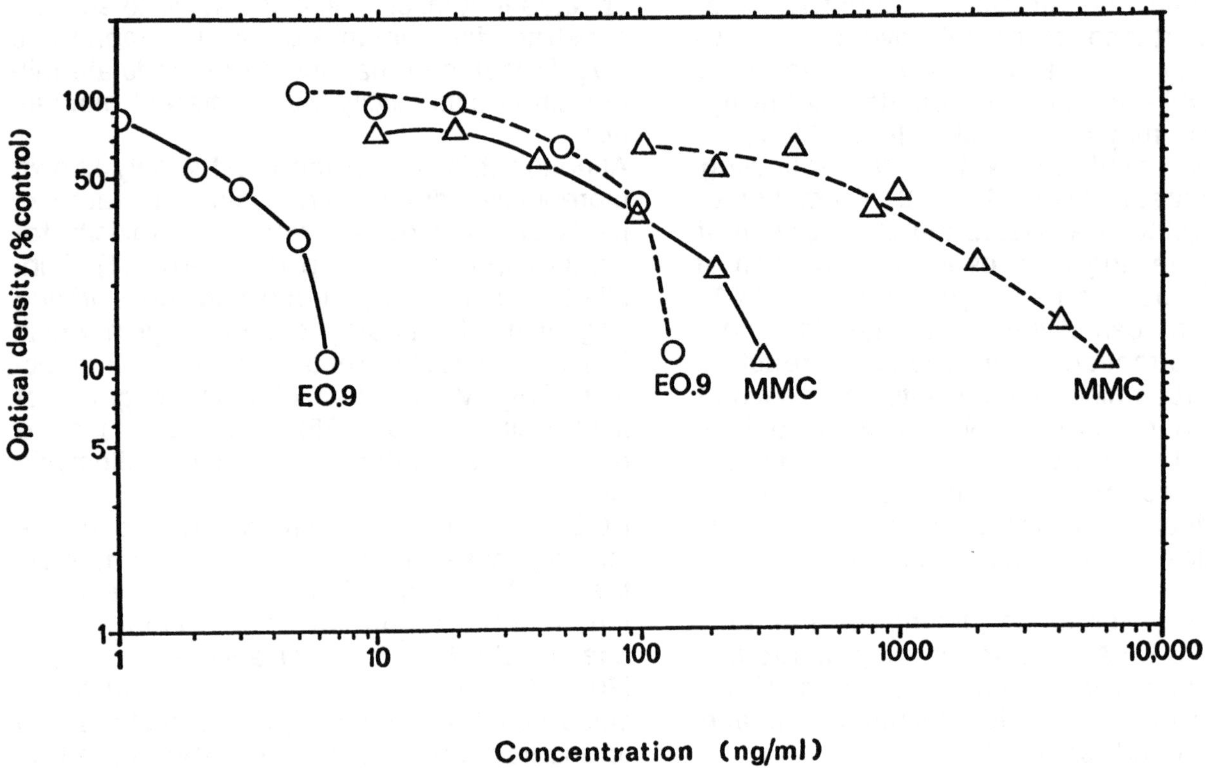

Fig. 17. Comparative toxicity of the novel indoloquinone E0.9 and mitomycin C (MMC) against EMT6 cells. Chemosensitivity testing was carried out using the MTT tetrazolium dye-reduction assay under aerobic conditions with 1h (broken line) or continuous (solid line) exposure. E0.9 is the more toxic under both conditions. Data from Kooistra KL and Workman P (unpublished)

Manipulation of Tumour Hypoxia

Studies are under way to determine the value of drugs which act to increase further the degree of hypoxia in tumours. Induction of extensive tumour hypoxia might have therapeutic potential in its own right, but will be perhaps most optimally applied in combination with bioreductive drugs [74].

An increase in tumour hypoxia can be produced by use of vasoactive agents such as hydralazine which act to divert blood flow from tumour to surrounding normal tissues via the "steal phenomenon" [74]. Such agents can markedly increase the antitumour effect of bioreductive agents such as SR 4233 [74], as well as conventional non-bioreductive alkylating agents such as melphalan [75]. This suggests a complex mechanism involving "trapping" the agent in the tumour, recently confirmed for melphalan (Stratford IJ and Workman P, unpublished), as well as increased bioreductive metabolism. In addition, the developmental agent flavone acetic acid has been shown to produce a marked and unusually prolonged decrease in tumour blood flow accompanied by an increase in tumour hypoxia [76]. This appears to occur through a novel mechanism, and experiments are in progress to assess the potential for combination with bioreductive drugs. Trapping of drugs together with induction of hypoxia can also be achieved using injections of microspheres for chemoembolisation in regional chemotherapy (see Noteborn and McVie, this volume).

Finally, induction of tumour hypoxia can also be brought about by agents such as BW 12C, which acts to increase the affinity of haemoglobin for oxygen [77], and by sudden changes in haematocrit level [78].

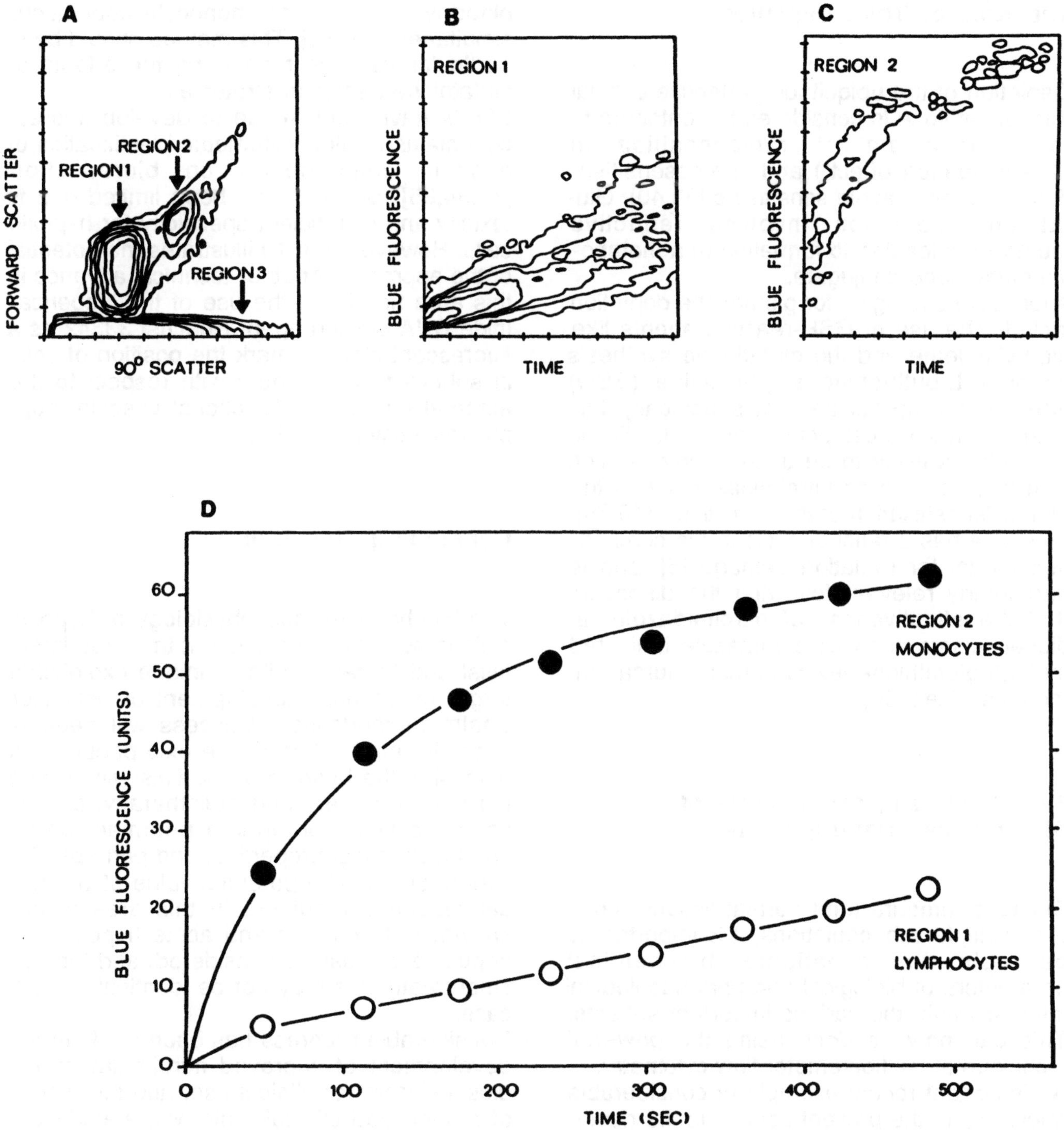

Fig. 18. Glutathione metabolism in human peripheral blood lymphocytes and monocytes assayed simultaneously by flow cytometry with monochlorobimane. The lymphocyte-enriched preparation was obtained from heparinised whole blood of a normal subject using Ficoll-Paque. Cells were mixed with 120 µM monochlorobimane at time zero. Lymphocytes (90%, Region 1) and monocytes (10%, Region 2) were identified in the 2-dimensional frequency contour plot of forward versus 90° scatter (A). Region 3 contained cell debris. Electronic gates were set around Regions 1 and 2 to obtain 2-dimensional frequency contour plots of intracellular GSH-monochlorobimane adduct fluorescence versus time (B and C). Median fluorescence is plotted against time in panel D. It can be seen that monocytes were more intensively stained than lymphocytes, consistent with larger amounts of GSH and/or GSH S-transferase. A total of 50,000 cells were analysed. Data from Workman P, Cox H and Watson JV (unpublished)

The Role of Thiol Depletion

Depletion of the ubiquitous protective cellular thiol glutathione is considered to contribute to the mechanism of radiosensitisation ("preincubation effect") and chemosensitisation by nitroimidazole sensitisers [33,40]. Glutathione depletion involves reductive metabolism leading to formation of a metabolite-glutathione conjugate.
Alternative strategies for glutathione depletion include the use of GSH-reactive agents like diethylmaleate and the glutathione synthesis inhibitor L-buthionine sulphoximine (BSO) [40]. These agents are not specifically targeted to hypoxic cell populations, but BSO in particular is likely to be used in combination with agents such as nitroimidazoles with the aim of "sensitisation of the sensitiser" [40,79]. This idea has a rational basis in the competition model for radiation damage [5], and is particularly relevant following the discovery that the effectiveness of nitroimidazole radiosensitisers such as etanidazole is limited by high glutathione levels in many human tumour cell lines [80].

Flow Cytometry for Analysis of Biochemical Heterogeneity

Because tumours (and normal tissues) contain multiple subpopulations, it is important to be able to investigate biochemical parameters of biological and pharmacological interest within the various important subsets. This can now be done using the powerful technique of multiparameter flow cytometry.
An important recent example of considerable relevance in the present context is the development of monochlorobimane as a fluorescent probe to study glutathione metabolism [81]. The fluorescent conjugate is formed between the probe and cellular glutathione, through the action of glutathione-S-transferases. Thus both these parameters can be studied with the technique [82,83]. As an example, Fig. 18 shows the ability to discriminate the glutathione content in peripheral blood lymphocyte and monocyte populations simultaneously [83]. This method should be of particular value in monitoring the effects of glutathione depletion strategies.
Efforts have been made to develop fluorescent stains for flow cytometric identification of hypoxic cells based on bioreduction [78,84,85]. Success has been limited due to toxicity and insufficient specificity for hypoxic cells. However, Fig. 19 illustrates the potential of the approach. Another technical advance in this area has been the use of the bisbenzamide DNA binding agent Hoechst 33342 as a fluorescent stain to mark the position of cells in spheroids or tumours with respect to the external medium or functional vascular supply, respectively [86,87].

Concluding Remarks

The biochemistry and physiology of hypoxic cells in solid tumours present the experimentalist and therapist with a unique exploitable target for rational development of optimised treatment modalities. Success will depend upon the eradication of the oxic populations alongside the hypoxic ones. This will involve the use of surgery and radiotherapy, as well as drugs with appropriate pharmacological and biochemical properties, and perhaps also hyperthermia. The potential value of biological response modifiers in this area is unknown. Both chronic and acute hypoxic cell populations must be considered, and the optimal treatments may not be identical in each case.
Considerable progress has been made in the development of improved nitroimidazole radiosensitisers for clinical use, and the results of randomised clinical trials with etanidazole and pimonidazole are awaited with interest. Optimisation of the structure and activity of mixed-function DNA-targeted sensitisers holds considerable promise. It appears possible to modify the molecular features of chemosensitisers so as to concentrate upon the pharmacokinetic modulation or the hypoxic cell targeted bioreductive mechanism as appropriate.

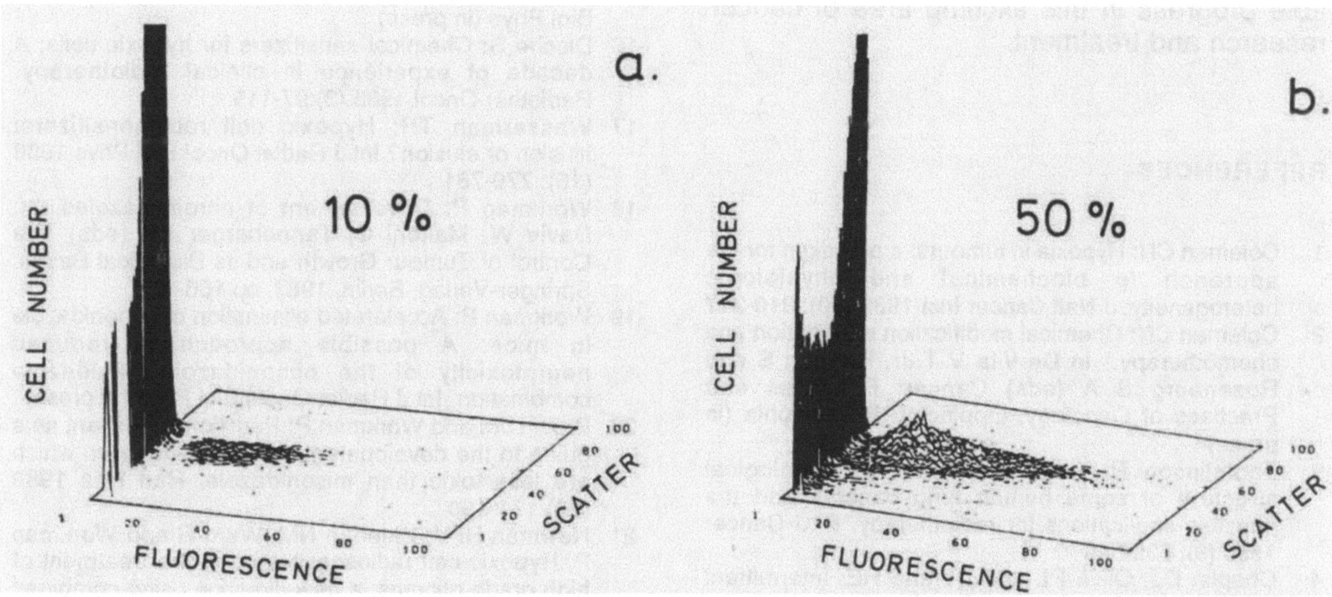

Fig. 19. Identification of hypoxic versus oxic cells based on reduction of a nitroacridine stain to a fluorescent product. Oxic and hypoxic cells were mixed after previous incubation with Nitroakridin 3582 (8 μM, 3h). The data are shown as isometric plots of fluorescence vs forward scatter (a function of cell size) vs cell number for mixtures containing 10% (a) or 50% (b) hypoxic cells. The hypoxic cells ("islands") are clearly separated from the oxic cells ("cliffs"). Reproduced with permission from Begg et al. [85]

Bioreductive drugs designed for preferential activation in hypoxic regions of tumours continue to be developed, and new classes such as the indoloquinones and benztriazine-di-N-oxides are of particular current interest alongside the mixed-function agents. The use of such agents together with hypoxia-inducing drugs including blood flow modifiers is under evaluation. Potentiation of bioreductive metabolism by therapeutic hyperthermia seems feasible. Coadminsitration of glutathione-depleting agents, particularly BSO, may be of special value with the nitroimidazole sensitisers.

The importance of elucidating the molecular enzymology of bioreductive activation pathways for particular compounds has been emphasised. An important goal is the rational selection of the appropriate bioreductive drug according to the individual patient's tumour biochemistry and physiology. The choice of drug may be altered in response to changes in these parameters during treatment, for example if a particular bioreductive enzyme is down-regulated while another is up-regulated.

Modified expression of bioreductive enzyme genes may be obtained using biological response modifiers. Improved assays for these enzymes for use on biopsy material would be valuable. Antibody and nucleic acid probes are likely to prove important tools, as will the development of improved flow cytometry technology for the multiparametric analysis and purification of multiple cell populations within heterogeneous tissue specimens. Fluorescent stains are becoming available for an enormous range of biochemical parameters. Important examples of flow cytometric probes include monochlorobimane for glutathione, fluorescent bioreductive markers for hypoxia and bioreductive enzymes, and Hoechst 33342 as a marker of proximity to functional vasculature.

Efforts will be redoubled to develop and evaluate various techniques to determine the number and location of hypoxic cells in human solid tumours. As well as the flow cytometry approaches mentioned above, interest will focus on non-invasive magnetic resonance spectroscopy techniques, particularly using ^{19}F-nitroimidazoles for imaging spectroscopy.

The next few years will surely see considerable progress in this exciting area of cancer research and treatment.

REFERENCES

1 Coleman CN: Hypoxia in tumours: a paradigm for the approach to biochemical and physiologic heterogeneity. J Natl Cancer Inst 1988 (80): 310-317

2 Coleman CN: Chemical modification of radiation and chemotherapy. In De Vita V T Jr, Hellman S and Rosenberg S A (eds) Cancer: Principles and Practises of Oncology. Lippincott, Philadelphia (in press)

3 Thomlinson RH and Gray LH: The histological structure of some human lung cancers and the possible implications for radiotherapy. Br J Cancer 1955 (9): 539-549

4 Chaplin DJ, Olive PL and Durand RE: Intermittent blood flow in a murine tumor: radiobiological effects. Cancer Res 1987 (47):597-601

5 Hall EH: Radiobiology for the Radiologist. New York, Harper and Row, 1978

6 Workman P: New drugs against hypoxic cells. Cancer Topics 1983 (4):54-55

7 Heacock CS and Sutherland RM: Induction characteristics of oxygen regulated proteins. Int J Radiat Oncol Biol Phys 1986 (12):1287-1290

8 Rice GC, Hou CA and Schimke RT: Transient hypoxia enhances the frequency of dihydrofolate reductase gene amplification in Chinese hamster ovary cells. Proc Natl Acad Sci USA 1986 (83):5978-5982

9 Chapman JD: The detection and measurement of hypoxic cells in solid tumours. Cancer 1984 (54):2441-2449

10 Franko AJ: Misonidazole and other hypoxia markers: metabolism and applications. Int J Radiat Oncol Biol Phys 1986 (12):1195-1202

11 Horowitz M, Blasberg R, Molnar P, Strong J, Kornblith P, Pleasants R and Fenstermacher J: Regional (^{14}C) misonidazole distribution in experimental RT-9 brain tumors. Cancer Res 1983 (43): 3800-3807

12 Urtasun RC, Chapman JD, Raleigh JA, Franko AJ and Koch CJ: Binding of ^{3}H-misonidazole to solid human tumors as a measure of tumor hypoxia. Int J Radiat Oncol Biol Phys 1986 (12):1263-1267

13 Raleigh JA, Miller GG, Franko AJ, Koch CJ, Fuciarelli AF and Kelly DA: Fluorescence immunohistochemical detection of hypoxic cells in spheroids and tumours. Br J Cancer 1987 (56): 395-400

14 Raleigh JA, Franko AJ, Treiber EO, Lunt JA and Allen PS: Covalent binding of a fluorinated 2-nitroimidazole to EMT6 tumors in BALB/c mice: Detection by F-19 magnetic resonance at 2.35 T. Int J Radiat Oncol Biol Phys 1986 (12):1243-1245

15 Maxwell RJ, Workman P and Griffiths JR: Demonstration of tumor-selective retention of fluorinated nitroimidazole probes by ^{19}F magnetic resonance spectroscopy in vivo. Int J Radiat Oncol Biol Phys (in press)

16 Dische S: Chemical sensitizers for hypoxic cells: A decade of experience in clinical radiotherapy. Radiother Oncol 1985 (3):97-115

17 Wasserman TH: Hypoxic cell radiosensitizers: Illusion or elusion? Int J Radiat Oncol Biol Phys 1988 (15): 779-781

18 Workman P: Development of nitroimidazoles. In: Davis W, Maltoni C, Tanneberger SE (eds) The Control of Tumour Growth and its Biological Bases. Springer-Verlag, Berlin, 1983, pp 166-172

19 Workman P: Accelerated elimination of pimonidazole in mice: A possible approach to reduced neurotoxicity of the pimonidazole-etanidazole combination. Int J Radiat Oncol Biol Phys (in press)

20 Brown JM and Workman P: Paritition coefficient as a guide to the development of radiosensitizers which are less toxic than misonidazole. Rad Res 1980 (82):171-190

21 Newman HFV, Bleehen NM, Ward R and Workman P.:Hypoxic cell radiosensitezers in the treatment of high grade gliomas: a new direction using combined Ro 03-8799 (pimonidazole) and SR 2508 (etanidazole). Int J Radiat Oncol Biol Phys 1988 (15): 677-684

22 Coleman CN, Halsey J, Cox RS, Hirst K, Blaske T, Howes AE, Wasserman TH, Urtasun RC, Pajak T, Hancock S, Phillips TL and Noll L: Relationship between the neurotoxicity of the hypoxic cell radiosenstizer SR 2508 and the pharmacokinetic profile. Cancer Res 1987 (47):319-322

23 Dennis MF, Stratford MRL, Wardman P, Watts ME: Cellular uptake of misonidazole and analogues with acidic or basic functions. Int J Radiat Biol 1985 (47):629-643

24 Dische S, Saunders MI, Bennet MH, Dunphy EP, Des Rochers C, Stratford MRL, Minchingon AI and Wardman P: A comparison of the tumour concentrations obtainable with misonidazole and Ro 03-8799. Br J Radiol 1986 (59):911-917

25 Stratford MRL, Dennis MF, Watts ME and Watfa RR: Radiosensitizer-DNA interactions. Br J Radiol 1988 (61):861-862

26 Roberts JT, Bleehen NM, Walton MI, and Workman P: A clinical phase I toxicity study of Ro 03-8799: plasma, urine, tumour and normal brain pharmacokinetics. Br J Radiol 1986 (59):107-116

27 Saunders MI, Anderson PJ, Bennet MH, Dische S, Minchinton A, Stratford MRL and Tothill M: The clinical testing of Ro 03-8799 - pharmacokinetics, toxicology, tissue and tumour concentrations. Int J Radiat Oncol Biol Phys 1984 (10):1759-1763

28 Honess DJ, Wasserman TH, Workman P, Ward R and Bleehen N M: Additivity of radiosensitization by the combination of SR 2508 (etanidazole) and Ro 03-8799 (pimonidazole) in a murine tumour system. Int J Radiat Oncol Biol Phys 1988 (15):671-675

29 Bleehen NM, Newman HFV, Maughan TS and Workman P: A multiple dose study of the combined radiosensitizers Ro 03-8799 (pimonidazole) and SR

2508 (etanidazole). Int J Radiat Oncol Biol Phys (in press)

30 Adams GE, Ahmed I, Sheldon PW and Stratford IJ: RSU 1069, a 2-nitroimidazole containg an alkylating group: high efficiency as a radio- and chemosensitizer in vitro and in vivo. Int J Radiat Oncol Biol Phys 1984 (10):1653-1656

31 Walton MI and Workman P: Pharmacokinetics and metabolism of the mixed-function hypoxic cell sensitizer prototype RSU 1069 in mice. Cancer Chemother Pharmacol 1988 (22): 275-281

32 Horwich A, Holliday SB, Deacon JM and Peckham MJ: A toxicity and pharmacokinetic study in man of the hypoxic-cell radiosensitizer RSU 1069. Br J Radiol 1986 (59): 1238-1240

33 Sieman DW: Modification of chemotherapy by nitroimidazoles. Int J Radiat Oncol Biol Phys 1984 (10):1585-1594

34 Mulcahy RT and Trump DL: Clinical chemosensitization by misonidazole and related compounds: a critical evaluation. J Clin Oncol 1988 (6):569-573

35 Workman P: Chemosensitization of lomustine by misonidazole, benznidazole and RSU 1069. Cancer Treat Rep 1986 (70):1139-1141

36 Roberts JT, Bleehen NM, Lee FYF, Workman P and Walton MI: A phase I study of the combination of benznidazole and CCNU in man. Int J Radiat Oncol Biol Phys 1984 (10):1745-1748

37 Bleehen N M, Roberts J T and Newman H F V: A phase II study of CCNU with benznidazole for metastatic malignant melanoma. Int J Rad Oncol Biol Phys 1986 (12):1401-1403

38 Bleehen NM, Freedman L and Stenning S: Phase III study of CCNU with or without benznidazole for recurrent gliomas. Int J Radiat Oncol Biol Phys (in press)

39 Coleman CN, Carlson RC, Halsey J, Kohler M, Gribble M, Sikic BI and Jacobs C: Enhancement of the clinical activity of melphalan by the hypoxic cell sensitizer misonidazole. Cancer Res 1988 (48):3528-3532

40 Coleman CN, Bump EA and Kramer RA: Chemical modifiers of cancer treatment. J Clin Oncol 1988 (6):709-733

41 Lee FYF and Workman P: Modification of CCNU pharmacokinetics by misonidazole. A major mechanism of chemosensitization. Br J Cancer 1983 (47):659-669

42 Lee FYF and Workman P: Misonidazole and CCNU: Further evidence for a pharmacokinetic mechanism of chemosensitization and therapeutic gain. Br J Cancer 1984 (49): 579-585

43 Lee FYF and Workman P: Misonidazole protects mouse tumour and normal tissues from the toxicity of oral CCNU. Br J Cancer 1985 (51):85-91

44 Lee FYF, Workman P and Cheeseman KH: Misonidazole and benznidazole inhibit hydroxylation of CCNU by mouse liver microsomal cytochrome P-450 in vitro. Biochem Pharmac 1987 (36):1349-1355

45 Workman P, Lee FYF, Walton MI, Roberts JT and Bleehen NM: Nitroimidazole inhibition of mouse and human cytochrome P-450 mediated hydroxylation of the chloroethylnitrosourea, CCNU. In: Benford DJ, Bridges JW and Gibson GG (eds) Drug Metabolism - from Molecules to Man. Taylor and Francis, London, 1987 pp 303-308

46 Hinchcliffe M, McNally NJ and Stratford MRL: The effect of radiosensitizers on the pharmacokinetics of melphalan and cyclosphosphamide in the mouse. Br J Cancer 1983 (48):375-383

47 Randhawa VS, Stewart FA, Denekamp J and Stratford MRL: Factors influencing the chemosensitization of melphalan by misonidazole. Br J Cancer 1985 (51):219-228

48 Horsman MR, Evans JW and Brown JM: Enhancement of melphalan-induced tumour cell killing by misonidazole: An interaction of competing mechanisms. Br J Cancer 1984 (50): 305-316

49 Murray JC, Randhawa V and Denekamp J: The effects of melphalan and misonidazole on the vasculature of a murine sarcoma. Br J Cancer 1987 (55):233-238

50 Lee FYF and Workman P: Nitroimidazoles as modifiers of nitrosourea pharmacokinetics. Int J Radiat Oncol Biol Phys 1984 (10):1627-1630

51 Kennedy KA: Hypoxic cells as specific drug targets for chemotherapy. Anticancer Drug Design 1987 (2):181-194

52 Zeman EM, Brown JM, Lemmon MJ, Hirst VK and Lee WW: SR 4233: a new bioreductive agent with high selective toxicity for hypoxic mammalian cells. Int J Radiat Oncol Biol Phys 1986 (12):1239-1242

53 Hewick DS: Reductive metabolism of nitrogen-containing functional groups. In: Jakoby WB, Bend JR, Caldwell J (eds) Metabolic Basis of Detoxication: Metabolism of Functional Groups. Academic Press, New York, 1982

54 Walton MI and Workman P: Nitroimidazole reductive metabolism: Quantitation and characterization of mouse tissue benznidazole nitroreductases in vivo and in vitro. Biochem Pharmac 1987 (36):887-896

55 Walton MI, Wolf CR and Workman P: Molecular enzymology of the reductive bioactivation of hypoxic cell cytotoxins. Int J Radiat Oncol Biol Phys (in press)

56 Heimbrook DC and Sartorelli AC: Biochemistry of misonidazole reduction by NADPH-cytochrome c (P-450) reductase. Mol Pharmac 1986 (29):168-172

57 Knox RJ, Friedlos F, Roberts JJ: The activation of CB 1954 (2, 4-dinitro-5-aziridinyl benzamide) in Walker cells is by bioreduction to DNA crosslinking agent. Br J Cancer 1988 (58):252

58 Walton MI and Workman P: Pharmacokinetics and bioreductive metabolism of the benztriazine-di-N-oxide hypoxic cell cytotoxin SR 4233 in mice. Cancer Res (submitted)

59 Laderoute KR and Rauth AM: Identification of two major reduction products of the hypoxic cell toxin 3-amino-1,2,4-benzotriazine-1,4-dioxide. Biochem Pharmac 1986 (35):3417-3420

60 Laderoute K, Wardman P and Rauth AM: Molecular mechanisms for the hypoxia-dependent activation of 3-amino-1,2,4-benzotriazine-1,4-dioxide (SR 4233). Biochem Pharmac 1988 (37):1487-1495

61 Powis G, Hodnett EM, Santone KS, Lee See K and Melder DC: Role of metabolism and oxidation reduction cycling in the cytotoxicity of antitumour quinoneimines and quinonediimines. Cancer Res 1987 (22):2363-2370

62 Bachur NR, Gordon SL, Gee MV and Kon H: NADPH-cytochrome P-450 reductase activation of quinone anticancer agents to free radicals. Proc Natl Acad Sci USA 1979 (76):954-957
63 Tomasz M, Lipman R, Chowdary D, Pawlak J, Verdine GL and Nakanishi K: Isolation and structure of a covalent cross-link adduct between mitomycin C and DNA. Science 1987 (235):1204-1208
64 Vingen BA and Powis G.: Pulse radiolysis of anticancer quinones: radical life times, reactivity with oxygen and one-electron reduction potentials. Arch Biochem Biophys 1981 (209): 119-126
65 Keyes SR, Fracasso PM, Heimbrook DC, Rockwell S, Sligar SG and Sartorelli AC: Role of NADPH-cytochrome C reductase and DT-diaphorase in the biotransformation of mitomycin C. Cancer Res 1984 (44):5638-5643
66 Keyes SR, Rockwell S and Sartorelli AC: Enhancement of mitomycin C cytotoxicity to hypoxic tumor cells by dicoumarol in vivo and in vitro. Cancer Res 1985 (45):213-216
67 Schlager JJ and Powis G: Mitomycin C is not metabolised by but is an inhibitor of human kidney NAD(P)H: (quinone-acceptor) oxidoreductase. Cancer Chemother Pharmacol 1988 (22):126-130
68 Fracasso PM and Sartorelli AC: Cytotoxicity and DNA lesions produced by mitomycin C and porfiromycin in hypoxic and aerobic EMT6 and Chinese hamster ovary cells. Cancer Res 1986 (46):3939-3944
69 Chakrabarty S, Danels YJ, Long BH, Willson JKV and Brattain MG: Circumvention of deficient activation in mitomycin C-resistant human colonic carcinoma cells by the mitomycin C analogue BMY 25282. Cancer Res 1986 (46):3456-3458
70 Kooistra KL and Workman P: Analysis and preclinical pharmacology of the indoloquinone E0.9. Cancer Chemother Pharmacol (submitted)
71 Powis G: Anthracycline metabolism and free radical formation. In: Powis G and Prough R A (eds) Metabolism and Action of Anticancer Drugs. Taylor and Francis, London, 1987, pp 211-295
72 Walton MI, Bleehen NM and Workman P: Heat-stimulated nitroreductive bioactivation of the 2-nitroimidazole benznidazole in vitro. Biochem Pharmacol 1987 (36):2627-2632
73 Walton MI, Bleehen NM and Workman P: Stimulation by localised tumour hyperthermia of the nitroreductive bioactivation of the 2-nitroimidazole benznidazole in mice. Cancer Res (in press)
74 Brown JM: Exploitation of bioreductive agents with vasoactive drugs. In: Fielden EM, Fowler JF, Hendry JH and Scott D (eds) Radiation Research. Taylor and Francis, London, 1987 pp 719-724
75 Stratford IJ, Adams GE, Godden J, Nolan J, Howells N and Timpson N: Potentiation of the anti-tumour effect of melphalan by the vasoactive agent, hydralazine. Br J Cancer 1988 (58):122-127
76 Eveloch JL, Bissery MC, Chabot GG, Simpson NE, McCoy CL, Heibrun LK and Corbett TH: Flavone acetic acid (NSC 347512)-induced modulation of murine tumour physiology monitored by in vivo nuclear magnetic resonance spectroscopy. Cancer Res 1988 (48): 4749-4755
77 Adams GE, Barnes DWH, du Boulay C, Loutit JF, Cole S, Sheldon PW, Stratford IJ, van den Aardweg GJMJ, Hopewell JW, White RD, Kneen G, Nethersell AB and Edwards JC: Induction of hypoxia in normal and malignant tissues by changing the oxygen affinity of hemoglobin-implications for therapy. Int J Radiat Oncol Biol Phys 1986 (12):1299-1302
78 Hirst DG, Hazlehurst JL and Brown JM: The effect of hematocrit on tumour sensitivity to X-rays. Int J Rad Biol 1984 (46):345-354
79 Kinsella TJ, Dobson PP, Russo A, Mitchell JB and Fornace AJ: Modulation of X-ray DNA damage by SR 2508 with or without buthionine sulfoximine. Int J Radiat Oncol Biol Phys 1986 (12):1127-1130
80 Phillips TL, Mitchell JB, De Graff W, Russo A and Glatstein E: Variation in sensitizing efficiency for SR 2508 in human cells dependent on glutathione content. Int J Radiat Oncol Biol Phys 1986 (12):1627-1635
81 Rice GC, Bump EA, Shrieve DC, Lee W and Kovacs M: Quantitative analysis of cellular glutathione in Chines hamster ovary cells by flow cytometry utilizing monochlorobimane: Some applications to radiation and drug resistance in vitro and in vivo. Cancer Res 1986 (46):6105-6110
82 Workman P and Watson JV: Flow cytoenzymology of glutathione metabolism. Cytometry 1987 (Suppl 1):270
83 Workman P, Cox H and Watson JV: Glutathione metabolism in human lymphocytes by flow cytometry. Cytometry 1988 (Suppl 2): 47
84 Begg AC, Hodgkiss RJ, McNally NJ, Middleton RW, Stratford MRL and Terry NHA: Fluorescent markers for hypoxic cells: A comparison of two compounds on three cell lines. Br J Radiol 1985 (58): 645-654
85 Begg AC, Engelhardt EL, Hodgkiss RJ, McNally NJ, Terry NHA and Wardman P: Nitroakridin 3582: A fluorescent nitroacridine stain for identifying hypoxic cells. Br J Radiol 1983 (56):970-973
86 Chaplin DJ, Durand RE and Olive PL: Cell selection from a murine tumour using the fluorescent probe Hoechst 33342. Br J Cancer 1985 (51):569-572
87 Olive PL, Chaplin DJ and Durand RE: Pharmacokinetics, binding and distribution of Hoechst 33342 in spheroids and murine tumours. Br J Cancer 1985 (52):739-746

Drug Delivery to Cancer Patients in Home Care: Experience with Intraarterial and Intravenous Chemotherapy

P. Schlag, A. Schwarz and S. Frohmüller

Section of Surgical Oncology, Department of Surgery, University of Heidelberg, 6900 Heidelberg, Germany

Rationale of the Project

Oncological therapy today is characterised by increased specialisation and concentration of therapy in tumour centres. In particular those patients who face long-term tumour-specific therapy are frequently hospitalised and therefore excluded from their usual psychosocial environment. For the tumour patient, this important additional burden means a substantially lowered quality of life. This problem is especially associated with continuous cytotoxic chemotherapy.

Because of this unsatisfactory situation we started an investigational project to transfer special oncological and supportive forms of treatment to the homes of the patients [1,2]. The aim of our study is to maintain the quality of life without diminishing the standard of tumour therapy.

Organisation of Home Therapy

In order to make cancer therapy possible on an outpatient basis, in November 1986 a team was set up at the Surgical Oncology Section of the Department of Surgery of the University of Heidelberg, FRG. It consists of two physicians, two nurses, and one psychologist. It considers itself a link between the hospital, general practitioner, community nursing services and patients and their relatives (Fig. 1). According to this concept, the team gives support to the patient, general practitioner, and the community nurses as well as to the relatives, so that the various types of oncological therapy that require special skill and knowledge can be carried out at home. The team is also in charge of instructing the patient in the specific treatment modalities that are mandatory for the realisation of home treatment. It is also important to become familiar with the patient's social surroundings. Only then can the therapeutic concept be aligned effectively with the patient's needs and the efforts of a standardised tumour therapy with a high standard of treatment. At the same time, it is expected that home treatment will contribute to lowering the costs of the health system. All the staff members work on a full-time basis and an additional stand-by service is available to the patients.

The team is financed by the authority for Social Affairs of Baden-Württemberg, FRG and collaborates with the Association of General Practitioners of Nordbaden, FRG.

The team's work is divided between the work at the hospital, where the team's office is located, and visits to the patients at their homes or at the general practitioner's office.

Coordination and documentation as well as preparation of the therapeutical apparatus and elimination of cytostatics etc. are performed at the office.

Following a training phase and consultation with the general practitioner the tumour-specific therapy is performed at the patient's home or at the general practitioner's office. Since the patients live within a radius of 100 kilometers, the visits are made by means of two passenger cars.

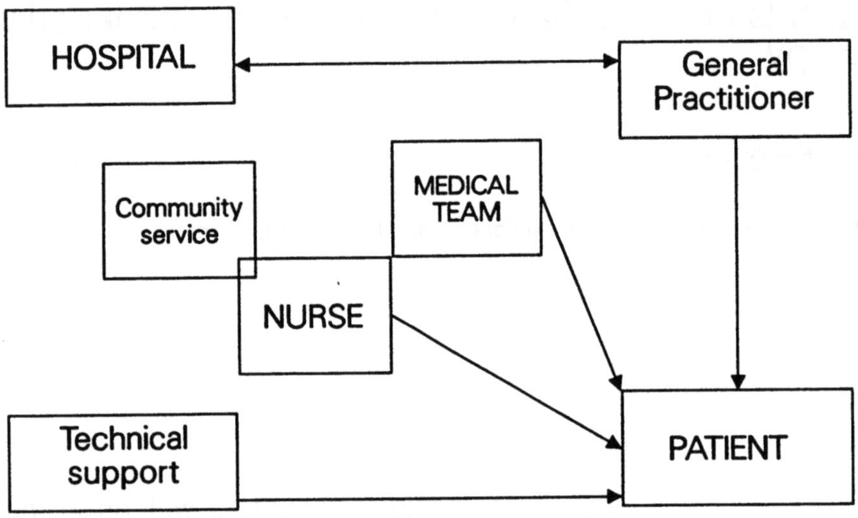

Fig. 1

Experience with Drug Delivery at Home

From November 1986 to August 1988 a total of 162 cancer patients, 97 male and 65 female with a median age of 59 years, were treated at home. Ninety-eight of these patients required enteral nutrition, wound care, or pain therapy. The remaining 64 patients with metastatic cancer received continuous chemotherapy at their homes after a training phase at the hospital. Thirty-eight of the patients had metastases of colorectal cancer in various organs. These patients were treated by means of continuous intravenous chemotherapy. Twenty-six patients had exclusively colorectal liver metastases. These patients were treated by hepatic artery infusion chemotherapy. The continuous chemotherapeutical infusions were administered via an implanted catheter system. Routinely, 5-fluorouracil was given in a dose of 1 g/m^2/day intraarterially or 650 mg/m^2/day intravenously per continuous infusion over 5 days. After 2 weeks of rest, the cycles were repeated.

The continuous cytostatic therapy was administered by means of portable pumps. A total of 394 cycles were administered, which is equivalent to 2,085 days of treatment at home. The team was responsible for carrying out the complete therapy cycles. The patients were visited regularly at home during treatment. Depending on their own initiative and degree of familiarity with the cytostatic treatment, the patients were supported or supervised individually, in cooperation with the general practitioner, in continuing the treatment.

The course and complications of the treatment were recorded and documented prospectively. Patients were also questioned by means of a semistructured interview at regular intervals in order to quantify their therapy tolerance and degree of satisfaction with life during the treatment. The continuous outpatient home treatment was terminated when medical reasons or technical problems contraindicated continuation of the treatment.

An in-patient learning phase proved to be important for a problem-free realisation of the home treatment since, firstly, this was the best way to familiarise the patients with the treatment form and, secondly, the treatment team was able to recognise the most urgent problems in the treatment of the individual patients.

The treatment of 15 patients had to be discontinued prematurely due to catheter occlusion. An extravasation in the area of the injection chamber occurred 24 times and was accompanied by transient local inflammation. As this subsided in all cases within a few days the therapy had to be interrupted only temporarily. No skin or subcutaneous necroses occurred after extravasation of 5-fluorouracil. Complications resulting in a postponement or delay of the therapy due to technical problems were therefore relatively rare (Table 1). Further side effects of the treatment were rare and consisted mainly of slight gastrointestinal complaints (Table 2).

Table 1. Reasons for termination/interruption of continuous chemotherapy (64 pts. 395 cycles of chemotherapy)

	Termination (% of patients)	Interruption (% of cycles)
Side effects		
Gastrointestinal	-	10 (2.5%)
Leukopenia	-	1 (0.2%)
Catheter complications		
Occlusion	9 (2,3%)	2 (0.5%)
Dislocation	6 (1.5%)	-
Infection	2 (0.5%)	-
Material breakage	1 (0.2%)	-
Paravasation	-	24 (6.1%)

Table 2. Side effects of continuous 5-fluorouracil chemotherapy (650mg/m^2 resp. 1000 mg/m^2 over 5 days) measured by WHO criteria

	Degree by WHO criteria				
	Degree 0	Degree 1	Degree 2	Degree 3	Degree 4
Haematological toxicity					
Leukopenia	87%	7%	7%	-	-
Thrombocytopenia	93%	7%	-	-	-
Gastrointestinal toxicity					
Bilirubin	97%	3%	-	-	-
Transaminases	63%	30%	3%	3%	-
Nausea/vomiting	47%	27%	17%	10%	-
Diarrhoea	93%	7%	-	-	-
Mucocutaneous	83%	7%	7%	3%	-

After some initial hesitation, the technical apparatus connected with continuous chemotherapy was accepted as a necessary matter of course, and in the end some patients were able to handle it autonomously. Psychological evaluation found that the possibility of home treatment enables the patients to maintain a satisfactory quality of life (Fig. 2). The most significant advantages for the patients were the avoidance of hospitalisation, the maintenance of family life, and the possibility to maintain occupational and recreational activities.

An inquiry among the general practitioners demonstrated the high level of acceptance of the mobile outpatient treatment. The concept was considered to be an advance in cancer therapy, profitable to the patient and in most cases a relief for the relatives.

The most important advances for the general practitioner were the steady availability of a competent colleague, the close cooperation, support and relief of the general practitioner and patient, the advanced training, and the lower costs of the entire treatment.

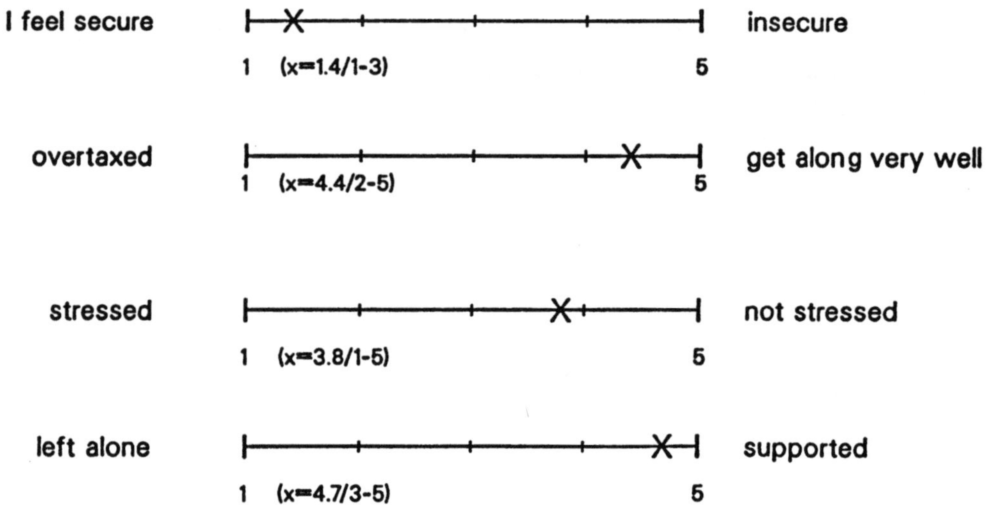

Fig. 2. Estimation of the momentary mood by the patient on a 5-point rating scale

The first results of a cost analysis show a reduction of about 50% compared to the costs of in-hospital treatment.

Conclusions

Experience with the transfer of in-hospital therapy forms to the outpatient sector exists in particular for continuous peritoneal dialysis [3,4] and total parenteral nutrition [5,6]. Particularly in the USA, increased efforts have recently been made to transfer special oncological therapy modalities also to the home [7]. However, it is not so simple to apply this directly to our system of medical care. Nevertheless, experience shows that in principle it is also possible in our case to transfer special oncological treatment to the outpatient sector, a prospect that certainly offers advantages for the patient. For the implementation of outpatient treatment the steady treatment team proved to be necessary and helpful for the patient.

The theoretical advantage of intraarterial or continuous intravenous chemotherapy in colorectal cancer is, apart from the direct administration of cytostatics in the intraarterially treated group, principally the reduction of systemic side effects [8,9].

In addition to the port systems we use, we have the choice of using fully implantable medication pumps for continuous chemotherapy [10,11]. In the latter case the treatment is certainly more comfortable than with continuous administration of drugs by means of external pump devices, but the therapeutic spectrum of fully implantable medication pumps is limited [12]. Essentially, only a 14-day continuous infusion with one cytostatic substance, namely 5-fluoro-2'-deoxyuridine (FUDR), is possible at present. This cytostatic treatment, however, has been questioned recently because of a substantial long-term toxicity [13,14]. Even when these aspects are taken into account, the course of treatment we pursue proves to be superior.

However, it is questionable as to what extent the survival time of the individual patient with metastatic colorectal cancer can be improved by means of available cytostatic treatment. It is all the more important, therefore, that efforts to improve the quality of life of patients receiving cytostatic treatment, as was attempted in the model described, should continue to be made.

REFERENCES

1 Ophof J, Leucht R, Frohmüller S, Doersam J, Ruoff G, Schlag P: Experiences in Home Care of Patients - A New Approach in Cancer Nursing. Acta Oncol 1988 (in press)

2 Schlag P, Frohmüller S, Ophof J, Leucht R, Doersam J, Ruoff G: Mobile ambulante Nachbehandlung (MAN). Münch med Wschr 1988 (130):284-288

3 Baum M, Powell D, Calvin S, McDaid T. McHenry K, Mar H, Potter D: CAPD in children comparison with hemodialysis. New Engl J Med 1982 (307):1537-1575

4 Moncrief JW, Popovich RP: CAPD update. Masson Publishing USA Inc. Austin 1981

5 Joyeux H, Solassol C: Ambulatory Parenteral Nutrition in Oncology. Bibl Nutr Dieta 1985 (35): 63-70

6 Reitz MV, Mattfeldt-Beman M, Ridley CM: Current Practices in Home Nutritional Support. Nutr Supp Services 1988 (8):8-14

7 Vinciguerra V, Degnan TJ, Sciortino M, O'Connell M, Moore T, Brody R, Budman D, Eng M, Carlton D: A comparative assessment of home versus hospital comprehensive treatment for advanced cancer patients. J Clin Oncol 1986 (4):1521-1528

8 Lokich J, Bothe A, Fine N, Perri J: Phase I Study of Protracted Venous Infusion of 5-Fluorouracil. Cancer 1981 (48):2565-2568

9 Schlag P, Hohenberger P: The Rationale of Intrahepatic Chemotherapy. This volume (1988)

10 Civalleri D, Cafiero F, Cosimelli M, Craus W, Doci R, Repetto M, Simoni G: Regional arterial chemotherapy of liver tumors. I. Performance comparison between a totally implantable pump and a conventional access system. Europ J Surg Oncol 1986 (12):277-282

11 Clark CG: Implantable vascular access devices in the treatment of colorectal liver metastases. Brit J Surg 1986 (73):419-421

12 Schlag, P: Continuous cancer chemotherapy - rationale and prerequisites for treatment at home. Int J Techn Assess Hlth Care 1985 (1):343-351

13 Kemeny MM, Battifora H, Blayney DW et al: Sclerosing cholangitis after continuous hepatic artery infusion of FUdR. Ann Surg 985 (202):176-181

14 Hohn DC, Rayner AA, Economou JS, Ignoffo RJ, Lewis BJ, Stagg RJ: Toxicities and complications of implanted pump hepatic arterial and intravenous floxuridine infusion. Cancer 1986 (57):465-470

U. Veronesi (Editor in Chief)

Surgical Oncology

A European Handbook

B. Arnesjø, L. Denis, F. Mazzeo (Co-Eds.)

1989. 224 figures, 226 tables. Approx. 1000 pages.
Hard cover. ISBN 3-540-17770-1

The European Society of Surgical Oncology and Springer-Verlag, Heidelberg, are pleased to announce forthcoming publication of an interesting and exciting new textbook for all those involved in oncology and related specialties: "Surgical Oncology – A European Handbook".
The first of its kind in Europe, this handbook has sought to cover most of the aspects of surgical oncology, which, with the recent moves toward a multi-disciplinary approach in research and treatment, every surgeon needs to know.
This handbook will be an essential feature of every surgeon's library. Dealing, as it does, with the many facets of the disease from biology of cancer, detection and diagnosis, general concepts, emergencies, rehabilitation and the planning and evaluation of therapy to the treatment of cancer of the different organs, it is a basic guide to the surgical approach to neoplastic disease.
Contributions have come from the most prestigious names in the European oncological world and will surely be a must in years to come – an invaluable reference for all those who have a specific interest in the field of oncology and the many and varied problems related to patient care and treatment.

Springer-Verlag
Berlin Heidelberg New York
London Paris Tokyo Hong Kong

Springer

European School of Oncology

ESO Monographs

Series Editor: U. Veronesi

L. Denis, Antwerp (Ed.)

The Medical Management of Prostate Cancer

1988. 8 figures. IX, 98 pages. Hard cover. ISBN 3-540-18627-1

B. Winograd, Amsterdam; **M. Peckham**, London; **H. M. Pinedo**, Amsterdam (Eds.)

Human Tumour Xenografts in Anticancer Drug Development

1988. 37 figures. XV, 143 pages. Hard cover. ISBN 3-540-18638-7

F. Cavalli, Bellinzona (Ed.)

Endocrine Therapy of Breast Cancer

Concepts and Strategies

1986. VII, 120 pages. Hard cover. ISBN 3-540-16959-8

F. Cavalli, Bellinzona (Ed.)

Endocrine Therapy of Breast Cancer III

1989. 26 figures, 7 tables. VII, 65 pages. Hard cover.
ISBN 3-540-50819-8

J. F. Smyth, Edinburgh (Ed.)

Interferons in Oncology

Current Status and Future Directions

1987. VII, 70 pages. Hard cover. ISBN 3-540-18019-2

L. Domellöf, Örebro (Ed.)

Drug Delivery in Cancer Treatment

1987. VII, 99 pages. Hard cover. ISBN 3-540-18459-7

A. B. Miller, Toronto (Ed.)

Diet and the Aetiology of Cancer

1989. 2 figures. VII, 73 pages. Hard cover. ISBN 3-540-50681-0

Springer-Verlag
Berlin Heidelberg New York
London Paris Tokyo Hong Kong

Springer

MIX
Papier aus verantwortungsvollen Quellen
Paper from responsible sources
FSC® C105338

If you have any concerns about our products,
you can contact us on
ProductSafety@springernature.com

In case Publisher is established outside the EU,
the EU authorized representative is:
Springer Nature Customer Service Center GmbH
Europaplatz 3, 69115 Heidelberg, Germany

Printed by Libri Plureos GmbH
in Hamburg, Germany